CANCER

FACTS & FALLACIES

By J. I. Rodale & Staff

Rodale Books, Inc.
Emmaus, Pennsylvania

Table of Contents

Part One: Cancer, Disease of a Thousand Causes

Part Two: The Accepted Treatments

Part Three: Treatments Not Officially Accepted

Part One:

CANCER, DISEASE OF A THOUSAND CAUSES

CHAPTER I

A Disease of Civilization

In 1957 the Pasteur Institute of Paris published a book in French entitled *Cancer—Nature, Cause and Cure,* written by one of its staff, Dr. Alexander Berglas, a book which was considered important enough to be published also in English. This book is honored with a preface by Dr. Albert Schweitzer in which he says that when he came to Africa in 1913 he saw no cancer cases there. "This absence of cancer," he says, "seemed to me due to the difference in nutrition of the natives as compared to the Europeans. The most significant difference being that the natives two hundred miles from the coast consumed no salt." Later when the natives began to use salt, "We have seen cases of cancer in growing numbers in our region. . . .Of my experience in Gabon, I vividly recall the 27th of April, 1954. That day we performed our first surgical operation for appendicitis on a black native. In 40 years we had

[3]

never had a diagnosis of appendicitis among these people. I have naturally been interested in any research tracing the occurrence of cancer to some defect in our mode of nutrition, and in particular in the most remarkable and original work of Alexander Berglas."

The theme of Dr. Berglas' book is that "the progressive artificialization of the environment of man—to which the human organism fails to adapt—may be an essential causal factor in carcinogenesis (cancer)." These are the words of Prof. Dr. Hans Lettre of the Institute of Experimental Cancer Research, Heidelberg, Germany. He states, regarding Berglas' work, "He further advances ideas that a cure of cancer must be possible by overhastening the division of the tumor cells. In numerous conversations we had discussed the question of the conditions under which such acceleration of cell division might lead to a loss in the vitality of tumor cells." This is a revolutionary concept. Instead of stopping the cells from multiplying, he wants them to multiply so fast that they will lose their vitality and burn themselves out, so to speak. But we are not going to concern ourselves with the curative speculations advanced by Dr. Berglas. We will devote ourselves to the "prevention" aspects of his book. It is that portion of his ideas we will concentrate on.

It is Dr. Berglas' contention that cancer is a healing attempt of the body brought on by chronic exposure to injurious agents whose action prevents the healing attempt from being completed; that cancer develops when the body's regulatory mechanisms fail; that irritation and deficiency factors will cause the regulatory mechanism to fail. He lists these factors as industrial injurious agents, denatured nutrition, artificial fertilizers, production of adulterated foods, accumulation of insecticides in foodstuffs, etc.

The author compares the cancer process to wound-healing, and finds that the two have a great deal in common. In cancer it is as if the body has incurred a wound and the cancer process is part of the attempt of the body to cure that wound. In other words, cancer is a curative attempt on the part of the body.

The author describes symbiosis, which means the living together or close association of two dissimilar organisms. "The enormous importance of the symbiosis between man and nature, which has come into being in the course of millions of years, cannot be too strongly emphasized. We live in total dependency upon nature, and could, for example, not go on living if the oxygen would not be liberated by plants from the carbon dioxide exhaled by us.

"If we consider modern artificial fertilizers from the point of view of symbiosis, we find that here the symbiotic situation has been strongly affected. It is to be noted that straight chemical fertilizers are employed at the expense of the natural soil flora. True, soil life is at first encouraged, but the exceedingly diverse microorganisms that must live on organic matter are progressively destroyed. It must be borne in mind that individual species of plants have bred their specific microflora valuable to themselves. It is beyond doubt that bacteria and plants are interdependent. The excretions of the roots and root hairs attract bacteria and

[5]

cultivate them. We should realize that today the natural fertility of the soil as such is being destroyed. Even if yield has been artificially increased, it has been at the expense of quality. The manifold life of the soil has been destroyed in its interaction and with it the marvelous symbiosis which had developed between man, plant and soil. This symbiosis between soil, plant and man has been disrespected; yet our organism is dependent on nourishment from the outside, and any disturbance of symbiosis outside our bodies has its effect within our community of cells."

Dr. Berglas then describes symbiosis as it exists in the human body. He says, "The community of cells making up the human organism must also be regarded as an extremely well organized symbiotic system. It is composed of an abundance of different types of cells, each of which has a certain function to perform. These different types of cells are members of the community. They are interdependent; if the cells of the blood fail to transport oxygen, if the cells in the mucous membrane of the stomach fail to produce gastric juice, if the cells of the liver fail to detoxify, then the other organs and cells will perish. Whether sensory or neural cells, connective tissue or muscle, all cells live in symbiosis with the other specialists of the community. They are individuals, but individuals dependent on other cellular individuals. Without this symbiosis of the individual organs our life would be impossible.

"Symbiosis in the human body is no different from any other symbiosis; if part of it breaks away and becomes independent, as in the case of cancer, then not only is order disrupted at the point in question, but the harmony of the whole is disrupted."

Then follows a discussion of all the known vitamins, describing their functions in the body, and a summary to the effect that if there are deficiencies of them, or if the quantitative proportion among the vitamins is wrong, there is an impairment of our defensive capacity. In such a case, he says, especially when an outside irritation is added in the chemical additives used in our foods, a disorganization of process in cell metabolism will develop. This means cancer. In other words, Dr. Berglas believes that a deficiency of vitamins plus the irritation factor from chemical food additives could produce cancer.

He especially singles out vitamin C, stating that it must be mentioned in connection with the cancer problem. He says that a vitamin C deficiency will cause a liquefaction of the intercellular cement substance (collagen) resulting in the disintegration of existing scar tissue; it prevents healing, which, he states, is "a preconditioning factor in cancerogenesis."

Dr. Berglas makes an amazing statement. He says, "In spite of the therapeutic value of synthetic vitamins in the treatment of certain diseases, one should not believe that the mere ingestion of the pure synthetic vitamins, even if identical in chemical structure to the natural vitamins, necessarily has the same effect on our body as the consumption of vitamins in combination with their natural concomitants. The latter are not to be dismissed as 'excess baggage,' but must be

[7]

thought of as the result of millions of years of evolution of optimal combinations."

Dr. Berglas states that the regulatory mechanism of the body is governed by the autonomic nervous system, which can be affected by vitamin deficiencies and which is dependent on nutrition.

There is a chapter devoted to civilization as it affects the menace of cancer. In it the doctor says that the more civilization has advanced, the farther we have come away from a natural diet. "Our present-day diet consists to a large extent of adulterated and denatured foods, from which the most precious essential factors have been removed by coloring, bleaching, heating, preserving, etc. . . . Increased mass production becomes indispensable, so that our soil is rapidly being exhausted, and we are almost exclusively dependent on artificial fertilizers, which in turn change the composition of the produce.

"Not only is damage done by deficiency in certain necessary constituents such as vitamins, trace elements, enzymes and auxins, but the interaction of these constituents has also been adversely affected through the industrialization of food production. When we speak of diseases of civilization, we are talking about diseases which, in many instances, could be corrected by proper diet. The progressive deterioration of the dentition in civilized man is one example of the effect of inadequate diet."

He refers to Dr. W. Kallath, a German who is internationally known, as saying, "Respect for the natural product is an indispensable requirement in the field of nutrition . . . Improper living and faulty diet constitutes a life-long preparation for cancer.

"Therapeutic efforts, made in certain countries to control cancer by improvement of nutrition and natural diet, are supposed to have had some success. In some cancer cases a low-salt diet with added fresh fruit juices, vitamins, enzymes, minerals, etc. was prescribed. It is reported that in a few hopeless cases, this procedure has resulted in subjective improvement."

He states that the National Research Council (U.S.A.) emphasizes that there is a direct relation between nutrition and cancer. He gives many examples of experiments with animals, and shows that in the northern parts of Sweden and Finland there is a condition of anemia, an acidity of the gastric juice, and atrophy of the mucous membranes of the mouth, all of which are symptoms of the precancerous stage. This condition is attributed to a diet low in iron and vitamins, as the people in these northern regions live mainly on canned meat and eat very little fresh fruit and vegetables.

A strong part of Dr. Berglas' book deals with the injurious elements put in our foods in the food factories. In this respect he says, "Certain *noxae* (injurious agents) have accumulated to an unimaginable extent and assumed a profound influence on our life. The extraordinary dangers to which human health is now exposed have been repeatedly pointed out by many scientists, but these warnings passed almost unnoticed." He quotes Dr. G. Schneck, of Germany: "It is of the nature and essence of industrial civilization

[9]

to be toxic in every sense. Poison is its hallmark, poison its ineradicable brand." Says Dr. Berglas, "The food we eat has, in a few decades, been so altered and contaminated with chemicals that every mouthful we consume contains some traces of harmful substances."

"Another source of danger," says Dr. Berglas, "are chemicals used on citrus and other fruits (such as DDT, ethylene gas, coloring matter, odor-intensifying agents and diphenyl) to protect the plant against pests, artificially ripen the fruit, save it from spoilage and to render it attractive to sight and smell. According to Druckrey, diphenyl may undergo a change of structure in the body that converts it into a possibly harmful substance.

"The number of such alien substances that are supplied to the body in food is extremely large. Our canned foods, for example, contain various additives such as sulphuric acid, benzoic acid and salicylic acid, potassium metabisulphite, hexamethylene tetramine, and others. Our meats and sausages are treated with sodium nitrate, our wines are sulphured, flour is bleached with substances such as chlorine, nitrogen trichloride, sodium persulphate, sodium perborate, benzoyl peroxide, etc. These substances cannot be described as biologically inert. In grain elevators, DDT and other agents are used to exterminate insects. It is no longer possible to get along without these insecticides, as trees, bushes and vines must be sprayed with stronger and stronger poisons against insect attack because the plants are increasingly losing their former natural powers of protection while the insects keep the

[10]

upper hand and become adapted to the poisons. These poisonous substances have already been identified in human fatty tissue and even in mother's milk. Other possible sources of danger are the chlorination of drinking water, the lead in the water pipes, and the cleansers and detergents with which we wash our dishes and utensils, traces of which are often left behind."

A few pages are then devoted to other cancer-causing agents in our environment, to the exhaust gases, smog and tobacco. And he says, "I would like to say that a detailed enumeration of the *noxae* to which we are exposed every day would fill a good-sized volume."

The book goes into statistics to show how cancer is alarmingly on the increase. "The increase manifests itself still more convincingly in a report by the National Cancer Institute, predicting that 32% of new-born children are expected to contract cancer during their lifetime." This means one in three. "These statistics on increasing cancer mortality support my assertion that everyone will be threatened with death through cancer, unless we put forth every effort to find a cure."

We disagree with one statement made by Dr. Berglas. He says, "We have to face the fact that a reversal of the so-called cultural advances of recent decades is impossible and I believe that my contention—that no one can protect himself from cancer under present-day conditions—will be more readily accepted."

We are fortunate to have this book, an official publication of the Pasteur Institute. This now can be added to a pronouncement made by Alexis Carrel in his book, *Man, The Unknown*. Dr. Carrell was connected with

[11]

the Rockefeller Foundation. He said, "Man is literally made from the dust of the earth. For this reason his physiological and mental activities are profoundly influenced by the geological constitution of the country where he lives, by the nature of the animals and plants on which he generally feeds. His structure and his functions depend also on the selections he makes of certain elements among the vegetal and animal foods at his disposal. The chiefs always had a diet quite different from that of their slaves. Those who fought, commanded, and conquered used chiefly meats and fermented drinks, whereas the peaceful, the weak, and the submissive were satisfied with milk, vegetables, fruits and cereals. Our aptitudes and our destiny come, in some measure, from the nature of the chemical substances that construct our tissues. It seems as though human beings, like animals, could be artificially given certain bodily and mental characteristics if subjected from childhood to appropriate diets."

Carrel also remarks: "It (the organism) is also affected by the deficiencies of the essential physiological and mental functions. The staple foods may not contain the same nutritive substances as in former times. Mass production has modified the composition of wheat, eggs, milk, fruit, and butter, although these articles have retained their familiar appearance. Chemical fertilizers, by increasing the abundance of the crops without replacing all the exhausted elements of the soil, have indirectly contributed to change the nutritive value of cereal grains and of vegetables. Hens have been compelled by artificial diet and mode of living,

[12]

to enter the ranks of mass producers. Has not the quality of their eggs been modified? The same question may be asked about milk, because cows are now confined to the stable all the year round, and are fed on manufactured provender. Hygienists have not yet paid sufficient attention to the genesis of diseases. Their studies of conditions of life and diet, and of their effects on the physiological and mental state of modern man, are superficial, incomplete, and of too short duration. . . ."

CHAPTER II

Chemicals and Cancer

What is the major cause of cancer? Professor E. Boyland speaking to Britain's Society of Medicine said, "Most of cancer in man, probably nine-tenths, is caused by chemical substances, the remainder being caused by viruses and radiation." He called the most glaring examples of environmental carcinogens excessive cigarette smoking, atmospheric pollution, industrial carcionogens affecting workers, and food additives, including artificial coloring matter and their carcinogenic potentialities. The *London Times* (Feb. 13, 1967) quoted Professor Boyland as saying, "Such colors come in intimate contact with millions of consumers of the colored foods," Then he continued, "The more sophisticated we become in our food habits and the more dependent we become on stored and packaged food, the greater the tendency to color our food."

The *Times* was reporting on a problem that has occupied scientists for more than a decade. In 1939, the International Union Against Cancer suggested that governments revise legislation regulating the toxicity of chemical food additives in light of the fact that they might be cancer-causing. When the Union met again in 1954 it stressed that cancer-causing substances must be considered in a different category from other poisons. For substances that poison temporarily we can set "tolerances"—that is, we can allow small amounts of these substances in food, assuming that, in such small quantity, they will be harmless. But, said the statement of the Cancer Congress, "No substance which, in tests at any dose level, induces any type of malignant tumor in any species of animal, can be considered innocuous to human health."

At another Union meeting in Rome in 1956 Dr. W. C. Hueper of the National Cancer Institute made some strong statements on the subject of chemicals in food and their possible relation to the increasing incidence of cancer in our country. Dr. Hueper listed 20 groups of suspected food additives and 17 groups of suspected food contaminants. Many of these, he said, have not been adequately investigated for their possible cancer-causing qualities. These include such common additives as dyes, thickeners, synthetic sweeteners and flavors, preservatives, shortenings, bleaches, oils and fats, antibiotics, estrogen, insecticide residues, soot, chemical sterilizers, antisprouting agents, wrapping materials, and radiation.

Dr. Hueper published a list entitled, "Environmental Cancer Hazards—a List of Causal Agents, their Occurrence in Industrial Operations and Products." The

[15]

substances listed by Dr. Hueper are those anyone might come into contact with every day. Chromium for instance. Here is a partial list of the processes in which workers come into contact with chromium: tanning, photography, paint, ink, textile, rubber, plastic glass, petroleum, blueprints, electrical appliances, drycleaning fluids, paint pigments, bleaching agents in fats and oils. That is only a partial list.

Residents in the vicinity of chromium plants, airplane manufacturing and maintenance establishments, railroad yards, shipbuilding plants, scrap metal smelters and oil refineries are all exposed to hazard. Then there are people who use home paints containing chrome pigments and chrome-containing anti-rust agents, and consumers of drinking water, polluted with industrial waste which contains chrome.

At the International Symposium of Medicine and Social Hygiene (September, 1957) Dr. R. A. Holman, a Welsh physician, said, "In my opinion, most of the chemicals added to food and drink for preservation or coloring could and should be abolished. The obvious way to preserve food is to make use of the energy provided by atomic power for deep freeze transportation and storage. This would insure a non-toxic food supply with many vital enzyme systems intact (assuming, of course, that the food stuffs are not covered or impregnated with toxic chemicals as a result of spraying, etc.)"

In 1961 there appeared the book, *Chemicals in Food and Farm Produce: Their Harmful Effects,* by Franklin Bicknell, M.D., consulting physician to the French

[16]

hospital, London, and co-author of a definitive work, *Vitamins in Medicine*. He wrote, "Probably few if any substances added to food are themselves capable of causing cancer. What the body turns them into is the danger. At present it seems possible that any dye is capable of producing cancer if it is broken down into certain substances by the body." The fact is that we actually know very little about such matters, even for a healthy human body, let alone one already disordered by liver trouble, menopause or transformed by pregnancy, etc. "While it is possible to show a diet dangerous, it is impossible to show that it is safe. It is not wise to eat any artificially colored foods, such as jams, iced cakes, sweets, ices, canned peas, margarine, custard powder, etc."

Any Dye Is Dangerous

What Bicknell is saying is that any dye is capable of causing cancer, depending on the way the body deals with it. Considering that dyes serve absolutely no purpose in food except to give it color it does not naturally have, there is a good argument against the Food and Drug Administration's permitting any dyes whatsoever in food.

In succeeding chapters Dr. Bicknell takes up preservatives and emulsifiers, flavorings, antibiotics, drugs, hormones, etc. "The daily consumption for many years of such meats (those treated with estrogen, a hormone) cannot be regarded with complete equanimity when it is remembered that synthetic estrogens are held to be related to leukemia and cancer."

[17]

Dr. Bicknell's basic premise in the book is that there is every reason, scientifically speaking, to believe that many of the substances now in food are terribly harmful. It is impossible to prove that they are not.

The U.S. Commission of Chronic Illnesses prepared a book entitled, *Prevention of Chronic Illnesses* (Harvard University Press, 1957) and in a chapter on cancer we find a three page list, in small type, of various substances *known to cause cancer*. Some of them are well known causes of cancer in human beings— arsenic and petroleum products. Other lesser-known substances have also been found to induce cancer in laboratory animals—dulcin (the artificial sweetener whose use in food is now forbidden) estrogens, DDT and certain dyes. Any one of these might appear in foods. Arsenic is widely used as an insecticide and of course DDT is too. Synthetic hormones are being used in meat animals, either injected or fed to them. Dyes occur in just about every processed food you buy. Nickel and chromium (both mentioned) contaminate food from metal containers. Carbon tetrachloride is another carcinogen, used to fumigate grain, and we have no way of knowing how much residue there is on the grain we eat.

To quote Dr. Hueper again, "The actual or possible existence of cancer hazards related to carcinogens in foodstuffs poses a serious public health problem, since the daily and life-long exposure to such agents would represent one of the most important of the various potential sources of contact with environmental carcinogens for the population at large, acting both on the

[18]

healthy and the sick, the metabolically normal and the abnormal alike."

Chemicals in food are there to profit the food processor; any service they might perform for the consumer is strictly incidental. It is the producer who makes extra money by extending the shelf-life of a product, by using a dye that gives his product better color than that of his competitor; a synthetic fat in the place of a natural one cuts costs for the producer, insecticides and fumigants cut down on spoilage losses. What does the consumer get? A potentially dangerous product he has been trained to demand, which is actually inferior to its unprocessed counterpart.

The question of cancer-causing substances in food was one of the most significant topics taken up at the Seventh International Cancer Congress held in London in July, 1958.

William E. Smith, M.D., director of Nutrition Research at Fairleigh-Dickinson University, brought the matter squarely to a head when he said, in his prepared address before the Congress: "Increasing knowledge of the ability of many different chemicals to incite cancer has, however, pointed to the need for tests extending over much longer periods of time, preferably over the full life-spans of test animals. It is, of course, now well known that a few doses, or even a single dose, of a carcinogenic (cancer-causing) chemical administered to a young animal can lead to development of cancer in middle life or in old age."

Does it surprise you to know that just one exposure

[19]

to a cancer-causing substance early in life can produce cancer twenty or thirty years later?

Dr. Smith went on to say that the peculiar long-delayed effect of these substances sets them apart from other chemicals which are just ordinary poisons. In the case of the latter substances, symptoms of poisoning appear rapidly and, if the person lives, he recovers from the experience with few ill effects. But with cancer-causing substances, there are usually no warning symptoms, yet the changes that occur in cells are irreversible and lead to cancer possibly many years later.

In 1939, Dr. Smith tells us, the International Union Against Cancer suggested that governments revise legislation regulating the toxicity of chemical food additives in the light of the fact that they might be cancer-causing. Later this Union established a committee on cancer prevention which, meeting in 1954, stated again that cancer-causing substances must be considered in a different category from other poisons. For substances that poison temporarily we can set "tolerances"—that is, we can allow small amounts of these substances in food, assuming that, in such small quantity, they will be harmless. But, said the statement of the cancer congress, "No substance which in tests at any dose level induces any type of malignant tumor in any species of animal can be considered innocuous (harmless) to human health."

Another symposium of the International Union was held in Rome in 1956. At this meeting Dr. W. C. Hueper of our National Cancer Institute made some very strong statements on the subject of chemicals in food and their possible relation to the increasing incidence of cancer in our country. The *New York Times* published a story about Dr. Hueper's speech in which he listed twenty groups of suspect food additives and seventeen groups of suspect food contaminants.

Meanwhile, the congressional committee to investigate chemicals in food held some hearings. Astonishing revelations were made before this committee as to the possible harm chemicals in food might be doing our people especially in relation to cancer. Congressman Delaney, chairman of the committee, introduced a bill in congress which includes provisions to (1) require testing of chemical food additives for their cancer-causing potential, and (2) forbid for use in food any additives that are found to be cancer-causing.

This seems to be a simple solution to the problem, doesn't it? And surely one on which everyone would agree! There cannot be an American food processor alive today so unfeeling as to knowingly cause cancer in any of his customers. Why then has the legislation been shelved? Why then do the years drag on with no regulations on cancer-causing chemicals in food, while at the same time the number of food chemicals is increasing every day? And the number of cancer deaths.

Complications Are Ever Present

Dr. Smith gives part of the answer in his statement before the Cancer Congress. Tests for possible cancer-causers are complex in the extreme. Certain substances may cause cancer under certain circumstances and may be highly beneficial foods under other circumstances.

[21]

For instance, sesame oil which had been heated to 350 degrees centigrade caused cancer in laboratory animals. Unheated oil did not.

Other aspects of the tests must be considered. Injecting certain substances may cause cancer while giving them by mouth may not. Substances which occur naturally may cause cancer when they are used out of context—that is, in other than natural ways.

Dr. Smith tells us that estrogen, a female sex hormone, is a powerful cancer-causer. Now obviously estrogen exists naturally in all females and does not cause cancer when it is performing its perfectly natural function of stimulating and regulating the various sex processes. But when estrogenic material from an animal is injected or given to a human being or another animal, it becomes cancer-causing. "The fact that some carcinogenic (cancer-causing) substances appear in nature is hardly a justification for extracting them and adding them to food," says Dr. Smith.

Finally—just what is a "safe" dose of anything which can produce cancer? Several years ago an insecticide was tested and it was found that laboratory rats got tumors when they ate this substance in relatively high doses. So a ruling went out that such and such a residue of this insecticide might appear legally in food. Later further tests revealed that cancer might be caused *at much lower levels* than the first experiment had shown. So the ruling was changed and no residue of that substance is now permitted in food.

How many people died of cancer because of that earlier erroneous ruling, do you suppose?

[22]

In closing, Dr. Smith tells us the unhappy news that what may cause cancer in one kind of animal may not do so in another kind. So tests with animals may show possible hazards for man, but cannot afford complete assurance of safety.

What Can We Do?

What is the answer for those of us who want to avoid cancer—and surely this means every one of us? Dr. Smith believes that, "In legislation to assure safety of chemicals in food, a conservative position would therefore be to limit artificial food additives to as small a list as possible sufficing to meet actual needs for production and distribution of foods." This is a very general statement of course and we wonder who is going to be the judge of what will "suffice to meet actual needs for production and distribution of food."

In a recent decision a certain dye was forbidden on Florida oranges because it has been found to be cancer-causing. But the citrus growers convinced the authorities that this dye was necessary "for production and distribution" of their product. It would be the ruin of the citrus industry if they could not dye their oranges, they said, so the dye is still being used. If this is the kind of decision such legislation will produce then it will be meaningless indeed.

We believe that legislation should be passed *outlawing all chemicals in food*. Certainly with today's provisions for refrigeration preservatives are never necessary. Dyes, thickeners, emulsifiers, bleaches, flavorings —all of these should be outlawed for good. Processed

[23]

food will look and taste a little different, true. Will the food companies lose money? Of course not, for the millions of dollars they are spending now promoting all these fantastic chemicals in foods they could spend in a grand, concerted publicity campaign to explain to the public just why and how such changes were made and what they will mean in increased health.

Don't you think everyone in this country would be delighted with such a prospect?

CHAPTER III

Are We Getting the Facts?

"Even governmental agencies are not legally authorized or morally entitled to permit, condone, or conspire
in the killing of people for private gain."

Those are the words of W. C. Hueper, M.D., in a
paper ("Cancer Hazards in Food and Consumer
Goods") he delivered in 1966 at the 11th annual convention of the National Health Federation. He went
on to point out that, authorized or not, government
agencies *are* collaborating in the sale of potential death
to the public.

Dr. Hueper retired in 1965 as Chief of the Environmental Cancer Division of the National Cancer Institute. Presumably he knows as much as anyone in governmental circles—and possibly as much as anyone in
medicine—about which elements in our environment
truly and actively threaten those exposed to them with
cancer. A prominent position in his Hall of Infamy is
occupied by synthetic chemicals.

[25]

"During the last century," he said, "the composition of the human environment, which heretofore consisted mainly of natural animate and inanimate factors, has been thoroughly revolutionized through the addition of a rapidly-growing number of new, and often synthetic, man-made chemical and physical agents.

"It has become increasingly evident during recent years that an alarming number of these new products are also potent poisons, or even cancer-producing agents, which have been widely disseminated in the human environment with foods, consumer goods and pollutants of the air, water and soil. As a result of rather common occupational and environmental exposures to these disease—and cancer-producing chemicals—often indiscriminately, if not unscrupulously, spread through the human economy—both production workers and the general public have become subject to new and serious health and cancer hazards.

"The cancer-producing, or carcinogenic, agents in this respect occupy an especially dangerous position, since their action is often insidious, for a long time is not accompanied by any distinct symptoms, and results in the appearance of cancerous growths many months, years, or decades after the first contact with such agents. For some of these carcinogens, an effective exposure may be relatively short and the amounts of carcinogens involved may be comparatively small; that is, they may not elicit any toxic reactions which may serve as a warning. . . . Observations made on experimental animals indicate, moreover, that carcinogens may penetrate the placental barrier and may be ex-

[26]

creted with the maternal milk and thus act upon the fetus and the infant.

"Although exposure to carcinogens in foods and consumer goods, like those present in air and water, is as a rule of relatively weak intensity, their actual or potential significance as sources of carcinogen risks is determined distinctly by the fact that they start early in life when the organism is most susceptible to their action, and that their contact often extends over 24 hours a day and over many years. The chances of their ultimate effectiveness in causing cancers have been improved during late decades. . . . It can be expected, therefore, that during the next decade a growing percentage of older individuals will respond with the development of cancers to exposures sustained during an earlier period of life."

Resistance and Harassment

Yet whenever Dr. Hueper attempted to do something about a terrible and worsening situation, he says, he encountered only resistance and harassment. "On several occasions," he says, "when circumstances required, i.e., when the papers submitted for clearance for publication dealt with carcinogens present in foodstuffs, the censors of the Public Health Service ganged up with those of the Food and Drug Administration.

"When in 1956 I submitted for clearance a paper on cancer hazards from food additives and contaminants, prepared for presentation at the Symposium of the International Union Against Cancer, held in Rome, I was advised by the information officer of the Public Health

[27]

Service that I should preface this rather lengthy and comprehensive discussion with the statement that the problems discussed were unimportant. My answer to this arrogant request was merely that I was not dull.

"At the same meeting, representatives of the Food and Drug Administration cited a statement of the Commissioner in which it was claimed that the American food supply was free from any carcinogenic additives and contaminants.

"The following carcinogenic chemicals present as additives, pesticide residues, and other contaminants have been discovered since then in American foods:

"The FD&C dyes yellow OB and yellow AB, which were shown in my laboratory to contain the potent bladder carcinogen beta-napthylamine, light green SF, brilliant blue, fast green, guinea green, estrogens, safrole, carboxymethylcellulose, aminotriazole, aramite, 8-hydroxyquinoline DDT, dieldrin, and arsenicals, in addition to distinct suspicions regarding petroleum waxes, Ponceau 3R (FD&C Red 1), sudan 3 (orange 3), orange SS (orange 4), oil red XO (red 14), orange II (orange 4), and citrus red #2."

In 1958 Dr. Hueper tried to obtain clearance for publication of another review on carcinogenic food additives—and failed. Says he: "Two years later the Secretary of HEW, Dr. Fleming, took action against the herbicide aminotriazole, because it was a carcinogenic contaminant of cranberry products." (Remember the sensation that caused?) "I submitted for clearance the same paper, greatly enlarged and provided with a new title. This time the article was approved within only

[28]

two weeks without any criticism as to its contents. It was then published in the *Archives of Pathology.*

"This experience," says the doctor, "is presented here as a striking example that the Public Health Service, when convenient for political reasons, has practiced unscientific censorship; and that evidently these efforts were successful by connivance of sufficiently and expendiently pliant so-called reviewing scientists."

Dr. Hueper concluded with the assertion that "there can be no compromise with the demand that the interest of the consumers, their health and life, should always and definitely be placed before the financial interest of industrial and commercial parties, and that this policy should be followed even when there is some uncertainty concerning the carcinogenic properties of a food additive or contaminant . . . Beyond any doubt, industrialization and chemicalization of the human environment not only will remain with us but will also in the years to come become more intense and more complex."

Certainly there should be no compromise by government agencies.

CHAPTER IV

Radiation and Leukemia

The death rate due to cancer increases year by year. And what are we doing about it? We are helping the rate to climb even higher. Why are we doing such a suicidal thing? Nobody really seems to know. It's not that we're not aware of what is happening, for respected scientists warn us about it every day. It isn't that we don't care, for we do care very much. When many of us read that more cases of cancer occur among children than any other disease, our emotions are certainly jolted. We are terrified at the thought of 11,000 new leukemia victims that materialize each year. But neither our knowledge and concern, nor our terror, seem capable of arousing any effective action on our part that would put a stop to this deadly game we play with such a consistent losing streak.

Once again from reliable, conservative sources, comes the warning that we'd better go slow on food additives, that we had better stop nuclear explosions until we know for certain that the consequences will not be tragically irreversible.

A Deadly Mix?

The Journal of the American Medical Association (April 11, 1959) calls our attention to the danger in which we place ourselves by manufacturing chemical substances outside of our biologic experience. By this is meant for example, the unpredictable substance that results when a housewife adds fluoridated water to a cake mix, bakes it in an aluminum pan, ices the cake with a prepared icing mix, and adds some coal tar coloring to top it off. Does the manufacturer of the cake mix, with its spoilage retardants and flavor controls, know for certain that artificial fluorides brought into contact with these ingredients in a stomach crammed with a hundred other chemical unknowns will not have a harmful effect? How could he? How could anyone who had not made careful and particular observations over a long period? Yet such cake mixes are sold—and bought—with not the slightest thought that such a product could be a main factor in our cancer record.

Dr. M. Burnet, whose writings in the South African *Practitioner* (no date) are referred to in the article, warns that we might unknowingly be producing substances which are capable of penetrating protective barriers which normally keep internal organs from contact with chemical substances that are capable of causing undesirable changes—poor eyesight or hearing, greater susceptibility to cancer, etc., if not in us, in

[31]

future generations. Dr. Burnet is referring, here, to radiation. This means radiation of all kinds—diagnostic X-ray, radioactive fallout, therapeutic X-rays, etc. We know full well that mutations, or changes like those Dr. Burnet mentions, can be caused to happen in animals by experimental procedures with radiation.

These irrefutable facts do exist: the cancer rate is rising; cancer can be caused by radiation; the nuclear explosions we have detonated have released more absorbable radiation in the years from 1945 to 1960, than was ever known in the world. Burnet says exposure to physical and chemical agents capable of causing mutations should be reduced as far as possible. Has any such thing been done? No, it is far down on the list, after first and second rate powers, preparedness, scientific advances, etc.

Leukemia Rate Advances

The incidence of leukemia (cancer of the blood that is almost always fatal) has been rising all over the world in our present century. In *The Lancet* (October 24, 1959) T. Alum Phillips, M.D., tells us that, in Britain, the leukemia rate in 1957 was five times what it was in 1920—a 500% increase! Dr. Phillips uncovered a few other statistical facts on leukemia: It is more prevalent in males than females; children and the aged are more affected than others; prosperous areas seem to be hit more frequently than those with a lower standard of living. Dr. Phillips' most startling revelation came from his comparison of figures on leukemia incidence in England for two four-year periods:

1950-53 and 1954-57. In the second period the leukemia rate increased 13%, and in some counties the increase was as high as 30 to 50%. At that rate of increase, can it be long before leukemia is as common as colds?

In the fourteen years since the first nuclear explosion in 1945, the leukemia count has increased in Britain by 150%, says Paul Mammet (*The Lancet,* November 14, 1959). After the infamous Windcastle nuclear reactor accident which caused the release of radioactivity over the territory, the nearby town of Seascale showed, that year, a leukemia death rate that was 36 *times the national average.*

A letter in *The Lancet* (November 14, 1959) from S. Lewin conceded that there is indeed a basis for concern, but urged that the geographical calculations of leukemia incidence are not as vital as finding a means for removing the leukemia-causing radioactivity which we find contaminating everything. He wants our scientists to work on finding a way to remove radioactive strontium from the milk we are drinking, and the water too, as well as from the grain and vegetables we eat every day. The problem is already with us and will be for many years, even if another nuclear explosion never occurs, so let's find a way to counteract it, says Mr. Lewin.

We think Mr. Lewin's view is an intelligent one. We think that some thought should be concentrated on dealing with the radioactivity we are already facing. We might be labelled prophets of doom to suggest that the radioactive elements in the atmosphere right now

[33]

are enough to annihilate humanity over a hundred or two hundreds years, but it is not impossible. Many scientists have said as much, after calculations which must, of necessity, be partly guesswork. But one guess is as good as another. We are dealing with a whole new entity. We can't predict what it will do to us, for we have no past experience for reference. Why not choose the safest course? We can do without atomic energy for a while longer. Let it be proven safe for living things, then everyone can relax while experiments go on. But this running at full speed in the dark, when at any moment one might plunge off a cliff, must seem the sheerest folly to any thinking person.

Leukemia is actually a disease of the organs which make the elements of the blood. However, it is identified in the minds of laymen as cancer of the blood, and the association is close enough to be considered applicable.

As explained in *Today's Health* (January, 1958), the body organs that manufacture the blood—the spleen, the lymph nodes, the liver and the bone marrow —"go on a frenzied spree, wildly producing white cells, many of which are abnormal, and reducing the elements needed for making red cells, and the tiny platelets that prevent and stop bleeding. . . . Overworking the blood organs to achieve this superproduction results in swelling and tenderness around the liver, spleen and lymph glands of the neck, armpits, chest, abdomen and groin. . . ."

The white cells, usually the body's defense against infection, are utterly inefficient in leukemia patients,

[34]

in spite of the great numbers of these cells which characterize the disease. Easy bruising and bleeding from delicate tissues in the nostrils and the gums occur because of the inefficiency of the platelets which are supposed to halt such bleeding or prevent it entirely. Because of the red cell supply being inadequate, the duty red cells perform, that of transporting oxygen to the tissues, is never fully accomplished. As a result, the leukemia patient grows progressively paler, more tired and short of breath.

The Types of Leukemia

Children are attacked most frequently by a type of leukemia known as lymphatic leukemia. When the white cells are immature the term "acute" is applied, and "lymphatic" leukemia means that the disease originates in the lymph glands. This type of leukemia has an extremely high mortality rate.

This same leukemia, when chronic (fully developed white cells), ordinarily strikes older persons, and, in them, is more benign than other types of leukemia. Conversely, myelocytic leukemia, a type of "adult leukemia" which has its root in the bone marrow, resists treatment and appears quite hopeless.

The accepted treatments for leukemia are radiation, blood transfusions and chemicals. None of these is presumed to be a true cure.

How Science Is Meeting the Challenge

A sad fact about the currently attempted treatment of leukemia is that the radiation and chemotherapy

[35]

which are held to be most promising are tied to the destruction principle. Instead of developing in the body a new strength which will help it to defend itself, these modes of therapy merely aim to destroy the leukemic cells. However, if the chemical or radiation dosage used is to be effective against the leukemia, it must also be so powerful that it destroys the ability of the bone marrow to manufacture blood cells. This being so such treatment can only end in death to the victim—if not from the leukemia, then from the treatment. Time is the only advantage to be gained. If the damaged bone marrow can manage to produce new blood fast enough to keep up with or surpass leukemic cells' survival rate, the patient continues to live, but as this ability diminishes, the patient weakens toward death. Unquestionably, since the very tool for survival —the bone marrow—is being attacked by the treatment, the cards are stacked against the patient. He might gain a few more months or so, but will not recover.

Bone Marrow Removed

An effort to evade what appears to be the inevitable lies in the work done by the New England Center Hospital and Tufts University Medical School. Experimentation there has aimed at a technique for removing a good part of the bone marrow while super doses of nitrogen mustard (deadly poison used as a leukemia treatment) are given to kill cancerous cells. Then the marrow is injected back into the patient after the series of treatments has been completed, the hope being that

[36]

the undamaged bone marrow will begin once more, once inside the patient, to manufacture wholesome red blood cells.

In an experiment with five patients described in the *N.Y. Times* (Feb. 22, 1955) the bone marrow was injected into the veins as described above. Three of the patients were said to have had brief remissions, but all five were dead as the report was made.

In the case of coritcosteroids used to treat leukemia, the destructive principle is again employed. Here the plan is to force acute leukemia blood cells into maturity and death by accelerating their old age, as it were. Leukemic cells are known to be slow to mature and hence have a greater staying power in the blood stream. They frequently divide before maturity, forming new, young, leukemic cells, and these never really grow old.

Cortisone used effectively to mature these cells is necessary in such great amounts that it will force the normal cells to maturity and death much faster than it can do so to the leukemic ones. *Science News Letter* (April 7, 1956) estimated the difference in speed in this way: "the normal cells start to show the effects of the hormone in about three minutes. The leukemic cells are not visibly affected for about 45 minutes." It is apparently another losing fight.

Methyl GAG Can Also Kill As It Cures

Methyl GAG is another of this type of therapeutic measure which can kill as it cures. In this case, Dr.

[37]

Emil Freireich of the National Cancer Institute, spoke with hope of leukemic remissions of from 4 to 14 weeks (*Drug Trade News,* November 13, 1961). The rub is that in patients with advanced neoplasms, clinical evaluation of methyl GAG revealed "impressive gastrointestinal and hemotological toxicity and in a few patients, severe hypoglycemia (low blood sugar)." A chemist producing the drug stated that the obvious goal is to produce similar drugs which would retain potency, but would have less toxicity.

A process which offered a different approach to the treatment of leukemia was reported in the February 22, 1955, issue of the *New York Times.* A Toronto, Ontario, doctor, Charles Bardawill, M.D., piloted a project which used a hormone extracted from the pituitary glands of hogs, sheep and horses. The treatment was intended, through the injection of this hormone, to correct the normal body supply of alkaline phosphate, thrown out of balance by leukemia. Dr. Bardawill's treatment fought to restore body processes to their normal function, rather than to destroy, by other means, the white blood cells produced uncontrollably by leukemia victims.

During a 10-day course of treatment with this method, the usual tests are reported to have shown a trend toward recovery of the patients. There is no indication as to how long the trend continued. However, this attempt at positive therapy has apparently been shortlived. The above described treatments are still preferred.

There is talk of a vaccine against leukemia, but the

[38]

very scientists who propose it are the first to admit that they are not sure what causes leukemia, and consequently can't be sure that a vaccine can be made, nor that it would be effective. Meanwhile the leukemia rate makes spectacular rises. The *New York Herald Tribune* (May 27, 1959) quoted the American Cancer Society as reporting a 300 per cent increase from 1930 to 1959. Only lung cancer has the edge on incidence and the hope of a cure for that disease is equally vague, it seems.

The Many Guesses

Guesses are numerous as to the actual cause of leukemia. *Scope* (November 19, 1958) headlined the proposition that a lack of an enzyme essential for normal growth is responsible when leukemia occurs. In the absence of this controlling enzyme a new and metabolically different race of cells grows. If this be true, the answer suggested by Dr. William Dameshek, Chief of Hemotology at New England Center Hospital, Boston, is to modify, somehow, the metabolism of these cells and to replace the missing enzyme. Apparently this job takes some time in the translation from theory to fact. Leukemia we still have with us, and no word since 1958 on the development of the missing enzyme or a means of modifying the metabolism of these cells.

In *Medical Science* (May 10, 1960) appeared Dr. Daniel Stowens' guess that diabetes and leukemia might be related. He found an insulin deficiency in the pancreas of leukemic children. Of 285 observed cases of leukemia in children, there was a 25 per cent inci-

[39]

dence of diabetes in the family (in contrast to only 4 per cent in non-leukemic children), and the presence of abnormal amounts of sugar in the urine.

Dr. W.J. McCormick wrote in the *Journal of Applied Nutrition* (volume 14, No. 1, 2) of his conviction that smoking by pregnant women is a factor in the rising rate of leukemia in children. In support of his contention, Dr. McCormick quoted two cancer workers, Lawrence and Donlan (*Cancer Research,* 12: 900-904, December, 1952) : ". . . The acute leukemias are an example of disease that may have such an origin (embryonic tissue damaged by carcinogenic agents). Leukemia seems to be increasing in recent years, especially in children under five years, suggestively due to carcinogenic stimulation in prenatal life."

Dr. McCormick believes that the carcinogenic factor mentioned is the neutralizing effect tobacco has on vitamin C. The fetus needs vitamin C and without it malformation of the blood-making system in prenatal existence is quite possible.

A short squib in *Today's Health* (December, 1961) told of a virus present in the blood streams of leukemic rats infected with what is termed "virus-caused leukemia." The question now is whether one can pinpoint viruses as the cause of human leukemia.

Some support of the virus theory appeared in the *British Medical Bulletin* (no date) where authors Stewart and Hewitt noted the very real increase in the leukemia rate and remarked that environmental factors must be considered. Virus is included among these.

[40]

Is It Modern Living?

A leukemia article which appeared in the *Chicago Daily News* (December 7, 1960) cited a study in New York State which seems to show that "the modern way of life has something to do with it (leukemia). It increases in families as economic standards increase." Does this point to increased luxuries (so-called) in diet for the children, such as more sweets, more highly processed foods? Does it point to a greater alcohol consumption, greater cigarette consumption in teenagers and adults? What do people who have enough money for more than the bare essentials do with it that might influence the blood manufacturing process?

The most likely of all guesses on the cause of the current rise in leukemia is radiation. It might be from therapeutic X-ray as well as from fallout after nuclear blasts. There are strong arguments which point to this possible cause as the most formidable one we will ever have to contend with. The *Journal of the American Medical Association* (January 16, 1960) carried a story which told of a survey of 6,473 children who had been given X-ray treatments since 1930, and "in agreement with previous investigations, the incidence of leukemia was higher among irradiated than among non-irradiated children."

Expectant mothers have long been warned against submitting to X-ray, especially in the pelvic area, either for treatment or diagnosis, unless there is a medical reason so urgent that waiting until the birth of the child is not practical. Much evidence has been pub-

[41]

lished in medical journals showing the link between leukemia in children, as well as other congenital defects in newborn babies, and prenatal use of radiation.

The Rise Is Worldwide

The rise in leukemia has been worldwide and Dr. Shields Warren, Professor of Pathology at Harvard Medical School, cited this rise as a possible result of greater radiation exposures all over the world. (*Scope,* February 12, 1958). Dr. Warren stated that he believed "there is a threshold of radiation necessary to produce leukemia . . . above 50 to 100 roentgens for adults . . . probably less for infants in utero (in the womb)."

Studies of cities in Japan which were bombed with nuclear explosives show that increases of leukemia have been induced by this radiation, according to Dr. Warren. He said that 2 per cent of those exposed to a single dose of 100 to 500 roentgens (a large amount) would become leukemic. He added that, ". . . there seems to be a wave of such leukemia 5 to 10 years after exposure."

There is no sure way to know if the genetic effects of radiation exposure due to fallout and direct exposure to nuclear explosions will afflict future generations with serious blood disorders until several generations have had time to be born. We do not know what dosage could have such effects. We do know that strontium 90, for one, is a radioactive element of fallout which seeks the blood-manufacturing bone marrow and can disrupt that entire process by the changes in the

[42]

cells it can cause. Increased fallout can only enhance the danger.

Are We Completely Helpless?

As we see the leukemia picture at present, the outlook is grim. One can only do one's best to avoid the suspected causes of this terrible disease, for once it takes hold, recovery through currently recognized medical implements is not very promising. Studiously avoid any unnecessary radiation, insure a generous calcium intake through calcium-rich foods and food supplements, including bone meal both as a decoy for Strontium 90 and a means of growing healthy strong bones; keep a high vitamin C level in the system, and eliminate the foods which are processed with possible leukemiogenic substances.

A Dangerously Narrow Attitude

Considering the admitted puzzle leukemia presents to medical researchers, we cannot suppress some irritation and dismay at the typical attitude of the medical men described in a story by Eldon Roark, which appeared in the *Memphis* (Tennessee) *Press Scimitar* (November 17, 1960). Mr. Roark told of a friend, Robert L. Miller, who was suddenly and seriously afflicted with leukemia. One diagnosis after another confirmed that fact. He was in a most critical condition, exhibiting some of the worst symptoms of leukemia.

Because he was so desperately ill, a new experimental drug was used on him—cyclophosphamide. In

[43]

10 days Robert was much better—well enough to go home. Once there he began to read about leukemia and became convinced of the value of diet in preventing a recurrence. He took to eating raw, fresh vegetables because, "Those writers convinced me that cooking destroys vitamins." He also ate plenty of meat. That, of course, was cooked.

Meanwhile he kept taking the cyclophosphamide pills along with a good diet. After 3 months he checked out as normal. The leukemia appeared to be gone!

The columnist friend was astounded by the story. He checked it out at the hospital. It was all true. Robert had had leukemia and it did appear to be arrested—the doctor wouldn't say "cured." Aside from the new drug, the doctor credited Robert's "attitude." He was unafraid. He kept working and remained cheerful.

"Yes, but what about the importance of raw vegetables?" asked the columnist of the attending physicians. "The doctors smile and shake their heads. They say Robert has become a food faddist. They don't think raw vegetables have played an important part in the case. 'Oh, food is important,' one of them said, 'you must have a balanced diet. But beyond that—' He shrugged."

How long Robert will continue to be well, we can't say. We can't say for certain whether it was the pills, the diet or both that brought him back to apparent health. But neither can his doctors!

How can they say with such assurance that diet was not a factor in his recovery? If cyclophosphamide were

[44]

solely responsible, there should be no talk of leukemia drugs being deadly and only mildly palliative. Here is a man who had the worst symptoms. He took a drug and the results were astounding. It was followed by a remission that had already lasted a year when the story was written. Why should researchers be fooling with bone marrow extracts if a drug they already have can do this!

We object to the doctors' slotting of Robert Miller in a food faddist pigeonhole because he began to eat raw vegetables. He believes that cooking destroys vitamins. Well, it does, and any of the doctors who snickered at his eating habits would have to give Robert right on this point. Furthermore, vitamins and minerals are essential to good tissues and bones—the tissues of the organs and the bones that make healthy blood. Is it faddism for Robert Miller to take the obvious precautions for saving himself from a relapse? We can only hope others stricken with leukemia, who are so fortunate as to have some improvement in their condition, will have the good sense to do the same. To those who are well and healthy we think Robert Miller's story may provide a good clue to a preventive course against leukemia's ever striking.

[45]

CHAPTER V

Danger in Every Breath

The evidence has convinced most people that smoking causes cancer; the evidence that auto exhaust in the atmosphere causes cancer should be equally compelling. Experts call the link statistical: cancer cases increase as the presence of auto exhaust increases.

Although there are many types of air pollution, the bluish haze that burps out of the tailpipes of idling automobiles, trucks, and buses in the center of your town is doing its share to hike the incidence of lung cancer as much as smoking or the air-borne wastes from the most irresponsible industries. Emission control devices to block these fumes are now required on new cars. How well they work and how much good they will do is problematical.

A public health research scientist, Dr. Eugene Sawicki, told a recent American Medical Association Medical Research Conference that compounds with the potential to change human heredity are found in pollution from automobiles and industrial plants. These

[46]

air-borne agents—"fairly prevalent" in the atmosphere of smoggy cities—are called mutagens, substances that cause mutations or changes in heredity. "We know these air-borne agents cause mutations in animals, but we made no test yet to determine the effect in humans. We have learned enough, however, to know that further investigation is warranted," said Dr. Sawicki.

The Sloan-Kettering Institute for Cancer Research developed a machine that breathed in air from a downtown New York street corner for six weeks. The tars were collected, then painted on the backs of mice. Ninety per cent of the animals developed skin cancer. Auto exhaust products contain three compounds closely linked to cancer, benzopyrene, aldehydes, and hydrocarbons.

The difference in cancer danger between auto exhaust and factory pollution was tested by Dr. Paul Kotin, Associate Director of the National Cancer Institute. He painted two groups of mice, one with auto exhaust tars and the other with tars from industrial pollution. One-third of the mice painted with auto exhaust residues got cancer. None of the other group was affected.

Lung cancer among males has gone up 1,900% from 1914 to 1950. According to *The N.Y. Herald Tribune* (April 5, 1966) Dr. Eugene Houdry, an authority on petroleum chemistry, reported that this increase "corresponds exactly" to the increase in gas consumption in the United States during the same years. The doctor also noted that lung cancer in males went down 35% from 1941 to 1945 when gasoline consumption was

[47]

reduced by exactly the same percentage because of World War II gas rationing.

The *Tribune* painted a picture any resident of a city with bus service would recognize at once: "The driver left the engine running, leaned back in his seat . . . unfolded his newspaper. The smoke and fumes from his diesel rose to blend with the exhausts of four other buses idling in the same short block." There is a law in New York against emitting smoke from any motor vehicle for more than ten seconds or leaving a stopped vehicle running for more than four minutes. The driver had his engine going for nineteen minutes. The law is rarely enforced in New York or in any other city that has such a law.

Wrapped in Fumes

The known cancer causers, as well as other poisons such as carbon monoxide and sulfur dioxide, are flung into the atmosphere every time an ignition key is turned even if emission controls reduce them. They contaminate the air for miles around the city. But people who live and work and even shop downtown are in particular danger. They cannot step out of a store or wait for a traffic light without being wrapped in cancer-causing fumes. They stand at a bus stop and suck in devastating exhaust from the buses and cars that pass as they wait.

Some people avoid downtown shopping for this reason. Some people have changed jobs and moved to small towns or to the suburbs rather than take their daily poisons. But some have no choice: they must maintain their jobs, so they must stay where the air is bad. And the cancer rate keeps rising.

[48]

CHAPTER VI

Pesticides Might Kill
You Too

There is no doubt that insects can be nuisances. Flies do buzz and show a distressing fondness for the top of one's nose, as well as for scheduling visits from the neighbor's garbage can right to your dinner table. Mosquitoes bite, wasps and hornets sting and ants invade the home by the thousands. Insects *are* nasty. But they aren't nearly as nasty as cancer of the liver.

Yes, it is cancer of the liver that a growing mass of evidence suggests is a likely sequel to the use over a period of years of many of the common household pesticides. An article pointing to exactly this danger and persuasively rounding up the evidence for it appeared recently in *Consumer Bulletin* (January, 1968).

Among other expert reports, the *Consumer Bulletin* article cited one that appeared recently in the *Archives of Environmental Health,* written by Dr. Hans L. Falk of the National Cancer Institute with Drs. Sandra J. Thompson and Paul Kotin. These three expert toxicologists, the article says, "Have called attention to a point which may be of great importance to the millions of consumers who use insecticides about the house and garden, or who have rugs, upholstery, or draperies that may have been treated with an insecticide. These researchers note that a limited number of the organic pesticides in common use today have been found experimentally to be carcinogenic in rodents used as test animals. They observed too that following high exposure to certain chlorinated hydrocarbons in food there were an increased number of liver tumors in rodents and certain kinds of fish. Commercial DDT had this effect in periods of exposure close to the life-span of test animals and was also found to produce liver cancer in rainbow trout when fed at 75 parts per million."

DDT Everywhere

DDT of course is one of the commonest insecticides in household use. Developed during World War II, at a time when newspapers and magazines made virtually no effort to distinguish between truth and propaganda, this nerve poison was widely reported to be deadly to insects but absolutely harmless to people. The completely false reputation for harmlessness persisted to the present day in the minds of many people. Until various government agencies began clamping down, restaurants would commonly spray DDT all around their

[50]

kitchens while butchers, bakers and vegetable dealers would heedlessly spray it on the foods they were selling in what they considered a sanitary effort to keep the bugs off.

How many people have been poisoned by such practices? Nobody knows. How many people are developing liver cancer today, or will develop it five years from now, because of the widespread and heedless use of DDT twenty years ago? Again, nobody knows. But when we finally find out, there is every reason to believe that the information will prove utterly shocking.

It is well known that all of us have inescapably been exposed to DDT. The poison has become omnipresent. It is in the water we drink, in the meat that we eat, in the milk we give our babies. The body accumulates and stores DDT in the fat, which represents a special menace to anyone who ever goes on a reducing diet. Sudden breakdown of large quantities of fat inevitably means the sudden release of large amounts of DDT into the bloodstream, where it might act as a nerve poison as it does on insects or stimulate development of cancer in the liver.

Another supposedly low-toxicity insecticide is pyrethrum, one of the most common in daily use. Regarding pyrethrum, *Consumer Bulletin* says:

"To increase its effectiveness . . . it is commonly associated in mixtures with a chemical substance known as piperonyl butoxide, which acts as a 'synergist,' a substance having a sort of booster action. Such insecticides are widely used on cocoa beans, stored grain (later processed into flour) and other foods to protect

[51]

against insect infestations. They are also applied to musk melons, tomatoes and other vegetables, and many fruits, *after harvest,* for the same reason.

"The scientists already mentioned note that the synergist action of piperonyl compounds is attributed to the inhibition of enzymes and consequently interferes with the detoxification actions which go on constantly in the human body. This interference with enzyme action leads to retention of poisons in the body, and accumulation of the toxic insecticide or its derivatives. (The liver detoxifies by changing a poisonous substance to a less poisonous one, or one that is more readily excreted.) The authors with great insight observed that an insecticide that interferes with the detoxification action of the body's organs may prevent detoxification of other potent organic substances to which man is exposed, and may thus be an indirect cause of cancer."

As Falk, Thompson and Kotin stated it in the *Archives of Environmental Health,* "Prevention of normal detoxification and elimination of the carcinogen introduces an additional hazard in the pathogenesis of cancer."

Piperonyl butoxide is chemically closely related to safrole, which is now banned from foods and drinks because it has been found to cause cancer of the liver and of the esophagus in rats. It has also been found in allied research to interfere with the elimination of benzopyrene, an extremely potent carcinogen present in cigarette smoke and indeed in the smoke of any of the fossil fuels such as oil or coal. It might simply be by making it harder for the body to eliminate benzopyrene

[52]

that piperonyl acts as a cause of cancer. But whether the causation is direct or indirect, it is certainly there. And every time you inhale some of the spray of a pyrethrum insecticide, or get some on your skin, or eat some on your food, you are taking some of this cancer-causing agent into your body.

Consumer Bulletin says that "Millions of persons suppose that because products to kill insects are freely sold and do not conspicously and strongly warn of their poisonous nature they must be without possibility of harm to users, and especially young children in the home. This belief is not warranted."

Naming only two as typical examples they go on to take a careful look at the labels of Raid House and Garden Bug Killer and Gulf Brand Aerosol Pesticide. The Raid spray contains .25 per cent pyrethrins, technical piperonyl butoxide .8 per cent, petroleum distillate 1 per cent. The Gulf Brand is reported to have a closely similar formula. Yet these pesticides are marked "Safe for humans, pets, foods when used as directed," on their containers.

Finally, *Consumer Bulletin* notes that a group of researchers at Harvard Medical School headed by Dr. Samuel E. Epstein has recently brought up a new aspect of the insecticide spray problem. "They showed that high levels of a combination of piperonyl butoxide and freon propellants as used in aerosol (spray can) containers have produced liver cancer when injected into mice."

The more we read, in fact, the more fully we agree with Dr. Deichmann of the University of Miami who

[53]

stated that "Sprayed pesticides are dangerous in any home. . . . Organic chlorine compounds, such as DDT and dieldrin are especially dangerous."

We're not very fond of bugs, believe us. But if we have to choose between bugs and pesticide sprays to get rid of them, we'll take the bugs anytime. Maybe it's old-fashioned of us, but we'd rather rely on good screens on our windows and the old fly swatter, put up with this annoyance of the bugs, and live to a ripe old age.

CHAPTER VII

Heated Fats Can Kill

Have you ever passed the exhaust fan from the kitchen of a restaurant? When you do, it is easy to detect the dominating odor of frying fats. These fats bubble and spit in deep fryers for days on end, without even a slight decrease in temperatures, which are held at 350° to 400°. When a customer orders fried chicken or fried shrimp or french-fried potatoes, with them he receives a free sample of the fat in which they were fried. This highly heated fat has been shown by some of our most prominent researchers to be a likely cause of cancer.

The distinction between highly processed or heated fats and natural ones is important. It would be wrong and dangerous to eliminate all fats from our diet. Our bodies need fats, and we number them among our most important foods. They are one of our best energy sources, offering nine times as much energy per gram as sugar does. Fats carry the B vitamin, pyridoxine and the fat soluble vitamins A, D, E, and K, which make fats vital to cell formation, especially cells of the

[55]

brain and nerve tissues. Finally, the body absolutely needs the unsaturated fatty acids contained in fats. These are indispensable in some processes of metabolism and cell structure. In high heats the vitamins A, E, and K are utterly destroyed. This vitamin destruction is illustrated by an experiment conducted by Dr. Lane and reported in the publication, *Cancer*, (Volume 3, 1950). A group of rats were mated for three years into seven generations. They were on a milk and white bread diet. After the second generation, a ration of lard heated to 350°, then cooled, was included in the rats' diet. From then on it was found necessary to feed the rats wheat germ oil and fresh vegetables prior to mating, because of the deficiencies in vitamins A and E caused by the pre-heated fats.

The use of heated fats by Americans is an insidious habit, so automatic that many health-conscious housewives include them in their menus without even being aware of it. For example, the lady who is so concerned for the health of her family that she wouldn't dream of serving deep-fried foods, can be found making a sauce from the drippings of a roast, quite unconscious that half of this liquid is fat that has been heated to 350° or more for several hours! Such fat has been made as hot as that used in the deep fryer—and it can be just as damaging.

Some Experiments With Heated Fats

In the periodical, *Cancer*, (Volume 3, #6, November, 1950), gastric (i.e. stomach) cancer is noted to be the leading cause of all cancer deaths, according to

[56]

statistics. Further, Dr. Geoffrey Hadfield, Dean of the Institute of Basic Medical Sciences, Royal College of Surgeons, has stated that cancer of the gastro-intestinal tract appears to be associated with a high fat diet. If this is the case, and if the body needs unprocessed fats as seen before, it is entirely logical that the processed, heated fats are the culprits in the case.

It is especially so when one reads that experiments with local applications of heated fats have shown tumors to develop at the site of the application. *The British Journal of Experimental Pathology* (Vol. 22, 1941) published data on experiments that resulted in cancerous lesions at the site of the injection in two out of twelve mice injected subcutaneously with cotton-seed oil which had been preheated to temperatures of 340°-360°C. When highly heated fats are brought into close connection with part of the body, apparently a weakness and predisposition toward cancer is introduced to that same part. It should be noted too that in the same experiment cottonseed oil heated to a lesser degree (200°-220°C.) did not produce any cancerous tumors in any of the experimental mice when injected in the same manner, leading to the conclusion that the dangers in fats vary in proportion to the heat applied.

In searching for clues to this highly heated fat and cancer relationship, a theory has been advanced by Dr. A. C. Ivy in *Gastroenterology* (March, 1955) which holds that hot fats reheated again and again undoubtedly increase the chance of producing carcinogenic substances. Obviously Dr. Ivy feels that there is a

[57]

dangerous change in the makeup of the fat each time it cools and is fired again, with the intensity of the heat of less importance. This should be a warning to housewives who save cooking fats for re-use.

A similar point of view shows up in the *Journal of Nutrition* (Vol. 55, 1955) in an article which discusses fats heated to relatively low temperatures (95°C.) and maintained at that heat for 200-300 hours. Refined cottonseed oil, heated thusly was included to make up 15 to 20 per cent of the diet of experimental rats. It was observed that rats on such a diet rapidly lost weight and died within three weeks. The loss of weight was accompanied by diarrhea and the occurrence of enlarged livers, kidneys, and adrenals and by shrunken spleens and thalamuses.

In spite of varying theories, the strongest suspicion for cancerous action of fats still seems to lie with fats that are preheated to a high degree, as witnessed by Lane and Associates and reported in the *Journal of the American Medical Association,* February 17, 1951. In an experiment, 5 rats were given regular rations of brown lard heated for 30 minutes at 350°C. Papillomas (tumors) of the forestomach and malignant tumors of the glandular stomach occurred in 37% of the rats, while similar symptoms were observed in only 5.7% of a control group which was fed unheated lard (though the fat was, of course, heated to make the lard in the first place).

For further data Dr. Lane injected 31 experimental rats with heated lard or vegetable oil. Three cancers developed in these rats, while none developed in a control group of 150.

A definite relationship between preheated fats and cancer showed up in a test discussed in *Modern Nutrition* for August, 1953, the official publication of the American Nutrition Society. A healthful, normal diet was fed to a group of rats. Then the rats were separated into two groups, and the normal diet continued, but for one addition: one of the groups was fed a daily ration of heated, hydrogenated fats, while the other group received a like amount of unprocessed fats.

After the eating pattern of this diet had been well established, a known cancer-producing substance, butter yellow, was introduced into the diet of all rats. Every one of the rats on the diet which included the preheated, hydrogenated fats developed tumorous growths, some of which proved to be malignant. The rats eating the unprocessed fats developed no tumors of any kind.

What Are Hydrogenated Fats?

Hydrogenated fats are everywhere. They come in cans and jars and cartons, looking as white and creamy as cold cream or yellow as the sun. They are guaranteed not to spoil, for there is nothing left in them that could spoil. And how did they get that way? They have been through about 18 different processes, including boiling, cooling, and boiling again, agitation, straining, catalytic action, bleaching, coloring, etc. Every life-removing process imaginable is applied to these fats. Most margarines are hydrogenated too and the false security bred by the idea that the margarines are

[59]

not made from animal fats but from vegetable oils is banished in an instant by this fact. Hydrogenation is what makes them spreadable and unmelting in summer temperatures, etc. They are as damaging to health as the frying and baking shortenings that are white and lardy-looking. Nor does the yellow color they are given, and the merchandising technique of presenting margarines in brick-shaped cartons make them as safe for you as "that other spread."

As seen by the various experiments noted here, it is still not generally agreed upon which heated fats do the most damage. Some say the danger lies only in fats heated to very high temperatures, others say it lies in fats heated and reheated, still another impression has it that fats heated for very long periods, even at relatively low temperatures, are the ones to watch out for. But one thing on which all of the experts agree—preheated fats can and may cause cancer! The investigation of treated fats in this connection is still a largely unexplored area. The explanation as to why these fats are antagonistic to our system has yet to be discovered, but the evidence of danger is clear enough to act as a warning.

We are convinced that the body welcomes the vegetable fats much more readily than the fats from animals. If there were no other reason, it is undeniable that most animal fats go through some processing before we get them. This may consist of cooking them at high temperatures in a roasting pan or broiler.

Of course the vegetable oils (especially those in unheated nuts, sun-flower seeds and so forth) have not been thus exposed and they are able to give the body what it needs without the risk of cancer that is lurking in heated fats. But even vegetable and cereal fats, once they are heated, may be cancer-causing.

How can you use this information practically in your kitchen? Does it mean that you should stop using fats altogether? Not at all. Here are some rules to follow if you would be absolutely certain you are not exposing your family to this particular risk so far as cancer is concerned.

First, never buy anything that has been fried. This means no potato chips, no roasted nuts, no frozen foods that have been fried or breaded and fried. Steer clear of anything fried in restaurants—fried clams, fish fillets, french-fried potatoes, fried eggplant, etc. Check closely with the waitress on any food where there is the slightest doubt.

By the same token, don't fry foods at home. This means don't do any frying at all, either in deep fat or in a frying pan. Any meat you would fry can be broiled just as successfully. And we advise removing the fat before cooking the meat, if you broil it, and also discarding the fat from roasts. Let's say you want to saute liver. A little vegetable oil—just enough to keep the meat from sticking to the pan—probably couldn't do any harm if you keep the heat low at all times.

Finally, don't buy hydrogenated shortenings (the solid kind) and don't ever, ever use drippings or oils over and over again. There is the risk of such fats being rancid, and of course there is the additional risk that they may be cancer-causing.

[61]

CHAPTER VIII

Cancer is Killing Kids

In 1962, cancer robbed about 4,600 children of life. The victims, all under 15 years of age, form a fatality list which surpasses the number of similar deaths only a decade earlier by nearly 30 per cent. An article in the *Statistical Bulletin* of the Metropolitan Life Insurance Company ("Recent Trends in Childhood Cancer," March, 1964), says cancer has for some time been the "leading fatal disease" in the 1 to 14 age group. At these ages, malignancies currently account for more than a fifth of all deaths from disease.

Upon examining the various types of cancer responsible for this frightening rate, the *Bulletin* reports that it is leukemia which claims "approximately half the total cancer mortality under age 15." Take a look at the statistics. From 1949 to 1951, leukemia rates per million for white boys from ages 5 to 9 and 10 to 14 were 38.8 and 26.4 respectively. Compare these data

[62]

to the time period from 1959 to 1961. Then, the rate per million for the first age group jumped to 49.0, and for the boys 10 to 14 years old, the rate per million went up to 31.0. For white girls in similar age brackets, leukemia mortality ran parallel to the boys' trends.

Some other major types of fatal cancer occur more frequently among boys than girls. Both lymphosarcoma (a malignancy arising in the lymphatic tissue) and Hodgkin's disease (a condition in which the lymphatic glands all over the body undergo progressive enlargement) strike boys more than twice as often as girls.

No Explanation

Apparently no one can explain why cancer is claiming so many victims so early in life. In recent years, it's the age group from 5 to 14 who have been hardest hit. In this group, boys (especially those from 5 to 9 years old) composed an appreciable increase in the death statistics. Their rates per million climbed from 82.1 (1949-1951) to 93.3 (1959-1961).

While cancer continues its rising importance as a cause of death among children in the United States, where can the blame be placed? Could there be any link between a cancer increase and an increase in the number of synthetics to which we are all subject? Just consider for a moment the ever-growing list of thousands of food additives and therapeutic and industrial chemicals that we must face every hour of the day. Sooner or later, won't these stimuli take their toll on us?

Perhaps Milton G. Bohrod, a physician from Roches-

[63]

ter, N. Y., provides a possible clue. In a letter Dr. Bohrod wrote (*Journal of the American Medical Association,* April 13, 1964), he points out that the body's capacity to react to these stimuli is limited to a relatively few ways. Dr. Bohrod believes that it is "reasonable to expect that many different combinations of environmental experiences may end up in a single final common pathway to which we give the designation: a disease."

The relationship Dr. Bohrod draws between these stimuli and disease makes good sense, for after all, how much can our bodies endure? Can the fact that more children are contracting cancer be one of the still unknown effects of the myriad potent chemicals we are forced to combine in our bodies with no knowledge of what they combine into, or what they do to us?

CHAPTER IX

Enzyme Poisons

A Welsh physician, Dr. R. A. Holman, believes he has the answer to the cause of cancer—and a stimulating and convincing theory it is, too. Dr. Holman, a bacteriologist, has spent the past 15 years studying cells —specifically the respiration of cells, how cells breathe. Although there is much that is still unknown in this field, it is apparent that there are at least three substances which are intimately involved in the process— oxygen, hydrogen peroxide and an enzyme called *catalase.*

Oxygen, as we all know, is important for every moment that we live. In fact, as Dr. Holman says in an article in *International Symposium of Medicine and Social Hygiene,* September, 1957, life *is* essentially respiration, or oxidation. But we also know that somewhere in the energy producing chain of events, oxygen reacts or combines with other substances to produce hydrogen peroxide.

[65]

Hydrogen peroxide is a poison to living tissue. So, obviously, if the process of life is to go on, something must be provided to counteract the possible harmful effects of hydrogen peroxide. A body substance, or enzyme, called catalase, has this function. It combines with the hydrogen peroxide, causing it to change into water and oxygen. So long as there is plenty of catalase in the cell to dispose of the hydrogen peroxide, all is well. But if something should cause more hydrogen peroxide to be present or if something should destroy the catalase in the cell, then we might expect trouble, for the hydrogen peroxide would be certain to do damage. As Dr. Holman puts it, "permanent changes may take place which will result in the genesis of malignancy."

If this theory is sound, it seems that those tissues which contain less catalase should be more susceptible to cancer than others. Investigators have found, sure enough, that those parts of the digestive tract where there is a smaller amount of catalase have a higher incidence of cancer than other parts of the digestive tract having larger content of the enzyme. The liver, where there is more catalase than any other part of the body, is rarely the site of primary tumors among people who have adequate diets.

We know, too, that the level of catalase is reduced in the liver and tissues of individuals with cancer. The faster the cancers grow, the greater the loss of catalase. One might think, therefore, that, in cases of cancer, you could simply give a preparation of catalase and the progress of the cancer would be arrested. But this

[66]

is not so, in the case of catalase. It seems that giving catalase once the cancer growth has started, causes the cancer cells to grow. The whole thing is, of course, another lesson in leaving well enough alone. We should not tamper with the delicate balance maintained at all times in the healthy cell. Naturally harmful substances can be handled by the body. It is only when we bombard it with manmade poisons that we run into difficulties.

What Substances Destroy Catalase in Our Bodies?

Dr. Holman tells us that barbiturates (sleeping pills) and various drugs for bringing down fevers (he does not mention these by name) have been cited as possible cancer-causers because of their action on this balance of hydrogen peroxide and catalase. The sulfa drugs also destroy catalase, thus adding to the risk of cancer. "During the past 15 years," he goes on, "millions of people have been subjected to the action of antibiotics. Most of these are very potent respiratory poisons, the exact nature of their action being, as yet, unknown."

Antibiotics are excreted rapidly from the body so perhaps they may not be as dangerous as they might be, but, he adds, no one knows how dangerous they may be when they are given in the form of long acting preparations, and over long periods of time. We think it is important to remember, in this connection, that much of our food contains antibiotics—milk, cheese, butter and meat because the animals involved have been fed antibiotics, whereas fresh produce and poultry are soaked in antibiotics to preserve them. What

[67]

other substances reduce the amount of catalase available to body cells, with disastrous results? Says Dr. Holman in the October, 1960, issue of *Mother Earth,* the journal of the Soil Association in England: "During the past 50 years many diverse chemical agents have been added to food and drink in order to kill bacteria, resulting in a longer shelf life. Most of these agents are potent catalase poisons. One of the main arguments in favor of adding chemicals is that this prevents much bacterial food poisoning in the consumers. This attitude, in my opinion, is over-stressed. It is not only the catalase content of the bacteria which is destroyed but also that of the food! This latter is an enzyme which is all-important for the prevention of cancer.

"In my opinion," Dr. Holman continues, "most of the chemicals added to food and drink for preservation or coloring could and should be abolished. The obvious way to preserve food is to make use of the energy provided by atomic power for deep-freeze transportation and storage. This would ensure a non-toxic food supply with many vital enzyme systems intact (assuming, of course, that the foodstuffs are not covered or impregnated with toxic chemicals as a result of spraying, etc.)."

It is also extremely important, Dr. Holman believes, that we take in as much catalase as possible in our food. This means eating as much raw food as possible, for enzymes (and catalase is an enzyme) are destroyed by heat. This fact alone must have a long-term effect on our health. "Cancer of the stomach is perhaps the commonest of our cancers," he says, "and yet we continue to ingest very hot materials coupled with calalase destroying chemicals. No other species of animal has such a diet. It would be to everyone's great advantage if the consumption of fresh, uncooked fruit and vegetables were markedly increased, thus ensuring a far greater catalase intake than hitherto in civilized populations."

Polluted Air is Part of the Problem

We inhale many substances which destroy catalase, he goes on. The vast amounts of various forms of sulfur which dirty our polluted air are catalase poisons. The fumes from our industries and our home heating units and incinerators, the deadly exhaust from trucks, and cars which pollute our highways, as well as the ever-present haze of cigarette and cigar smoke to which most of us are constantly exposed—all these are destructive of the important enzyme, catalase.

Dr. Holman mentions as extremely important, too, the aerosols containing insecticides, fungicides, antibiotics and so forth, which we use so extensively. We would add the many hair sprays used by women. The continued use of these over the years is what is dangerous for there is no doubt of the adverse effect they have on our cells, especially those of the respiratory tract.

This is what Dr. Holman has to say about oxygen: "A good oxygen intake is essential for good health. Totney would go so far as to explain the high incidence of cancer in the human race on the basis of poor or diminished oxygen consumption, and in a sense he is

[69]

right. Oxygen is essential for the removal and destruction of many toxic agents present on or in our cells, and it is, therefore, quite obvious that the more actively oxygenated our bodies the better we shall be able to combat the toxic agents which help to influence adversely our normal cells."

Finally, Dr. Holman warns us of the dangers of radiation. He protests particularly against the indiscriminate use of x-rays. At least, he says, we do not know where the threshold of safety lies in this regard or if indeed there is any level below which one can feel safe. No one can predict what will be the effect on the incidence of cancer 20 years from now of all the forms of radiation to which we are at present being exposed, he believes.

We think Dr. Holman's ideas, which have received wide and favorable notice from cancer researchers, are of the utmost importance. They provide yet another urgent reason for us to be ever alert to the dangers that surround us and eager to eliminate as many as we possibly can. Most of us cannot eat only food that has been organically grown and hence is free from all the poisons which are cancer-causing. But we can, certainly, buy food as fresh as possible. Dr. Holman's findings should add impetus to our letter-writing on the subject of chemicals in food—our protests to congressmen, to the newspaper editors, to boards of health.

CHAPTER X

Emotions May Have A Cancer Link

J. I. Rodale

In *The Sunday Observer* of England, January 22, 1967, there is a short article with the above title, and I am reproducing it herewith:

"In the past 10 years research workers have been considering the possibility that the mind, and especially the individual's emotional life may play a part in causing cancer, a disease which in this country claims 72 victims a day.

"For example, Dr. David M. Kissen, director of the Psychosomatic Research Unit, Southern General Hospital, Glasgow, investigated 366 patients suffering from lung cancer. Though there was little difference in the number of cigarettes smoked by the cancer patients and the control group, there was a marked difference in the personalities of the individuals concerned.

"Dr. Kissen found that lung cancer patients tended

[71]

to have poor emotional outlets. People who had adverse life situations and who repressed their feelings were more vulnerable to lung cancer than those who had good emotional outlets. Adverse life situations included disturbed marital relationships, poor relationships with parents and children, failure to gain promotion at work, and sexual difficulties.

"Strong supportive evidence for these findings was provided in a recent study undertaken by Drs. A. H. Schmale and H. P. Iker, of the Department of Psychiatry and Medicine at the University of Rochester Medical Centre, New York. Schmale and Iker selected 40 women who were known to have abnormal cells of the uterine cervix. They were interviewed the day after a definitive test for cancer had been made, but before the results of the test were known.

"The test took the form of an interview aimed at establishing the degree of hopelessness experienced by each patient. The interviewer then predicted on this basis whether or not cancer was likely to be present. This technique correctly identified eight out of 14 patients who had cancer, and 23 out of 26 who did not—an impressive result in statistical terms.

"Dr. Schmale says it is theoretically possible that the psychological reactions of these patients may be related to the preconscious or unconscious awareness of the presence of cancer in their own bodies. But it is equally possible that a life-history of endeavor coupled with a sense of hopelessness was a predisposing factor in the disease.

"None of these investigations implies that psycho-

[72]

logical factors alone are responsible for cancer, but they do suggest that there is some link between the disease and certain emotional states."

The above speaks for itself, and gives more evidence that cancer is less likely to strike happy people.

Dr. Denis Leigh

In the annual lecture of the Mental Health Research Fund, given in London, on November 1, 1966, Dr. Denis Leigh said the following, as reported in *The Lancet*, November 12, 1966:

"Epidemiological research had revealed illnesses in clusters related to life experience. Prisoners-of-war subjected to the harsh regimen of the Far East had more illness in later life than those who were in the European prison camps. Ex-prisoners of the Japanese six years later had twice the rates for cancer, heart disease, and suicide, and three times the rate for all forms of accident. These were not the diseases that would have been predicted. Inquiries in post-war Germany confirmed the pattern: Nazis dismissed from office had higher rates for all forms of illness than Nazis not dismissed."

The death of Jack Ruby, the slayer of Lee Harvey Oswald, fits into the pattern of this series. He died of cancer which induced a blood clot in his lungs. He had been a very unhappy man for a long time. Some people thought that his cancer was induced by feeding him cancer viruses, by mysterious interests that wanted him out of the way before another trial. But this is quite ridiculous.

[73]

Jack Ruby's death just adds another bit of evidence to our thesis that happy people rarely get cancer.

Another case is that of the "Oomph Girl," red-haired Ann Sheridan who died of cancer in January, 1967, at the age of 52. She had always been a stormy petrel, who was often suspended by the studios and would often go on strike for more money. Her life was a continuous struggle to go upward. She was married 3 times but never had a child. Ann Sheridan was too outgoing, too pushy.

There was a research at the Medical Research Council's Neuropsychiatric Research Unit, Carshalton, Surrey, England, which proved an earlier Swedish investigation that women who develop cancer are usually more extroverted, or outgoing in personality. In a study of 47 women, the results supported the idea that certain constitutional factors are associated with a predisposition of certain people to develop cancer. "Extraversion and other distinguishing factors may be related to physique and hormonal activity."

Our Experiment With Mice

In 1949, as president of the Soil and Health Foundation, I was associated with Dr. Ehrenried Pfeiffer in an experiment in the feeding of mice at his laboratory at Threefold Farms, Spring Valley, N.Y., the results of which were reported in *Bulletin 2 of the Soil and Health Foundation,* dated November 1, 1949. The experiment was undertaken in order to find out whether the treatment of soil with organic materials or with commercial fertilizers would show a difference in the

[74]

feeding and health value of products grown under such farming methods, and various groups of mice were fed by food raised by these different methods.

It was found that the death rate from fighting was distinctly higher in the chemical fertilizer group than in the organic one. There were more irritable and nervous mice in the chemical fertilizer group. I saw this for myself when I visited this experiment. The mice were kept six in a box and each box was divided into two rooms, because a mouse likes to sleep in one room and eat in another. In the partition between the two sections was a tiny door which was wide enough to permit one mouse at a time to walk through with comfort. When we opened up the chemically fertilized mouse box, that is, took off the top cover and let the light in, the mice became so frantic that they started to run. Two or three of them tried to go through the door at the same time, getting stuck and remaining there squealing and howling. But when we opened up the boxes in which the organically fed mice were kept, this did not happen. The mice continued nonchalantly about their business. It was interesting that the same thing happened time and again as we opened up the boxes. The chemically fed mice were invariably nervous while the organically fed ones were invariably relaxed.

Of the causes of death, stomach disorders were prevalent in the chemically fertilized group to an extent of about 16 per cent, but only about 3 per cent in the organic group. The results of this experiment showed that the survival rate of the organic group was mark-

[75]

edly higher than that of the chemical fertilizer group: 32.63 per cent as against 21.38 per cent in the first generation. In another strain of mice the survival rate was 64.41 per cent in the organic group as against 35.39 per cent in the chemical group. Large litters were born to the organically fed mice.

Some time later an interesting experiment was performed. It is a known fact that certain chemicals when rubbed on the skin produce cancer. One of these chemicals was applied to the skin of all the mice. On that of the chemically fertilized fed group, cancer of the skin reached as high as 71 per cent, but in the organically fed group only 45 per cent contracted it.

The organically fed mice were a very happy group, but not so the chemically fed ones. This experiment shows that good nutrition is a significant factor in developing a happy spirit.

Sir Robert McCarrison's Experiment

In 1927 when McCarrison was Director of Nutrition Research for India, he decided to find out if rats could be endowed with health equal to that enjoyed by the Hunzas, a remarkably healthy Pakistan people. He would do this by feeding the rats a diet similar to that consumed by the Hunza people. He divided his rats into 3 groups. One group was, consequently, fed the diet upon which the Hunzukuts and other healthy peoples of Northern India, such as the Sikhs, Pathans, and Mahrattas, subsist. Another group of rats was fed the poor diet of the Southern India rice-eaters, the Bengali and Madrassi.

[76]

A third group of rats was subjected to the diet of the lower classes of England, containing white bread, margarine, sweetened tea, a little boiled milk, cabbage and potatoes, tinned meats and jam. The results were startling. McCarrison described the first group as being *Hunzarized*. "During the past two and a quarter years," he stated, "there has been no case of illness in this 'universe' of albino rats, no death from natural causes in the adult stock, and but for a few accidental deaths, no infantile mortality. Both clinically and at post-mortem examination this stock has been shown to be remarkably free from disease of all kinds, including cancer, but the Bengali group of rats suffered from a wide variety of diseases which involved every organ of the body such as the nose, eyes, ears, stomach, lungs, bladder, kidneys, intestines, the blood, glands, nerves and reproductive organs. In addition, they suffered from loss of hair, malformed and crooked spines, poor teeth, ulcers, boils and became vicious and irritable."

The "English" rats also developed most of these troubles. They were nervous and apt to bite their attendants; they lived unhappily together and by the sixtieth day of the experiment they began to kill and eat the weaker ones amongst them. As you can see, the "English" rats were unhappy which seemed to be a concomitant of their ill health.

It would seem, therefore, that one step to being happy, and to be able to withstand the griefs and rigors of life, is to become extremely healthy. We want to make the health factor stronger than the unhappy factor.

[77]

The Work of David M. Kissen, M.D.
In Reference to Cancer of the Lungs

In the December 24, 1965 issue of *The Medical Officer,* there is an article by Dr. David M. Kissen, entitled "Possible Contribution of the Psychosomatic Approach to Prevention of Lung Cancer," which will be of interest in our study. It is based on a paper read to the Fourth International Conference on Psychosomatic Aspects of Neoplastic (Cancer) Disease at Turin, Italy, on June 10, 1965.

In this paper Dr. Kissen states that an effective preventive in cancer is based on the knowledge that cell changes precede the cancer perhaps by a considerable time; cervical smears, for example, effectively reveal precancerous conditions in cases of cancer of the cervix.

Dr. Kissen says, "An association between cigarette smoking and lung cancer has been substantiated so frequently as to lead to world-wide propaganda against cigarette smoking as a means of effectively reducing lung cancer mortality. Yet the long term effect in reduction of cigarette smoking is, by and large, slight. The cigarette smoker usually dismisses the propaganda as being applicable not to himself but the 'other guy' and the fact of the matter is that nine times out of ten he is right. Yet the minority are in danger and if advice against smoking could effectively be brought home to this minority many might well escape lung cancer. Would it not be a powerful contribution to prevention if one could identify these individuals who have a high risk of developing cancer so that preventive efforts may

[78]

be directed in the most economic ways? Likewise one could probably direct preventive efforts to the cancer-prone amongst women with negative cervical smears...

"On previous occasions (Kissen, 1963, 1964) I have described a personality characteristic that I found to be typical of lung cancer patients as opposed to non-cancer patients. The presence of this characteristic was elicited after 'blind' clinical appraisal of about 300 chest unit patients, half of whom were subsequently found to be suffering from lung cancer. The remaining patients served as controls. I described this character-istic as 'a poor outlet for emotional discharge.' This clinical observation was confirmed in a further series of over 400 chest patients, including more than 200 who were subsequently found to have lung cancer."

In other words, those cigarette smokers who had "a poor outlet for emotional discharge," were prone to get cancer of the lung. What does Dr. Kissen mean by a "poor outlet for emotional discharge?" I would take it he has in mind a person who is a more pessimistic type; who is a less happy person than one who has a good outlet for emotional discharge.

"As further confirmation a second control group was used. This comprised male non-cancer patients matched for age and social class from non-chest departments in the same hospitals. If one takes the non-cancer non-chest patients as representatives of the so-called general public, and the lung cancer patients as representa-tive of the general male lung cancer mortality, a sig-nificant relationship is found between lung cancer mor-tality and 'outlet for emotional discharge' (Table 1).

[79]

Those with a poor outlet have a lung cancer mortality rate of 270, those with a moderate outlet 112, and those with a good outlet 59. These figures are expressed per 100,000 per annum. The differences are present at all levels of cigarette smoking and among non-smokers as well as among pipe smokers. Put in another way, those with a poor outlet for emotional discharge appear to have more than four and a half times the mortality rate for lung cancer compared with those with a good outlet, and more than two and a half times the rate of those with a moderate outlet. Details of these findings are already published or in process of publication (Kissen, 1964, 1965). Here then is one feature of personality that may be used to help identify the lung-cancer-prone. It is worth remembering that this feature is similar to the independent description of repression reported by the Bahnsons (1964) in patients with cancers of varying sites."

TABLE 1

Lung Cancer Mortality Rates Per 100,000 Per Annum

	Emotional Outlet			All
	Poor	Moderate	Good	
Never smoked	50	11	—	23
Manufactured Cigarettes				
1-14 daily	260	66	38	93
15-24 daily	398	171	75	219
25 daily	452	176	132	243
Pipe only	59	26	33	44
All	270	112	59	145

Dr. Kissen gives some other psychological factors he found as a guide to lung cancer proneness. . . . Regarding this, he says:

"It is not just in the area of personality that psychological factors may be applicable in helping to identify the cancer-prone. Data that I have obtained, without knowledge of diagnosis, from more than 480 lung-cancer patients and 450 non-cancer control patients strongly suggest that certain environmental and social factors may contribute to the development of lung cancer. Such data may also be used to help identify those at risk for lung cancer. These data are at present being processed and will be published in due course. At this stage I can say that in the age group in which lung cancer is most frequent, the age group 55-64, and which in my series involves about 360 patients of whom more than half had lung cancer, evidence of serious environmental disturbances in childhood—especially inharmonious home and parental death—occurred with approximately similar frequency in the group of lung-cancer patients and the group of psychosomatic controls (controls with a history of defined 'psychosomatic disorder') and was twice as frequent in those two groups as among the remainder of the controls.

"Mention may also be made of the finding, in the same series, of the occurrence of significant long standing adverse situation in adult life in those men before the development of their cancer. This finding too has its potential use in identifying the cancer-prone."

In his summary Dr. Kissen advises preventive meas-

[81]

ures that could be concentrated on the cancer-prone minority. For one thing he would get them to stop smoking, and to use means to prevent children from starting the habit.

He says also that psychological care may be of value in preventing serious emotional results of major cancer surgery and other treatments. What he means, no doubt, is to encourage the patient to open up more, and to have a better outlet for emotional discharge. In other words to develop a more happy outlook on life. But this is rather late to change such an ingrown trait.

It would be better to start in schools, to have courses in how to cultivate a happy outlook, and to teach children how disease in general is quicker to attack unhappy people. There is much evidence of this. It is not only true of cancer!

The teacher should be able to pick out students that have a poor emotional discharge and try to cure them of this habit. An experience must be built up in this field.

An inhibited child grows up to be an inhibited, repressed adult, and it is these who commit suicide, who figure in divorces, and who get cancer more easily.

At the same time, the school as early as kindergarten should have means to teach children how dangerous smoking can be. The teacher can show how dirty the lungs become from tobacco, and in other ways appreciated by children, forever disgust them so that they will never begin this habit. As a Cardinal once said, "Give me the child until he is 6 years old and you can have him afterwards." Or was it 7 years? But whatever

[82]

it was, at an early age everlasting impressions can easily be established.

A Recent Study

It would be wrong to believe that modern science is entirely ignoring this intriguing question. Granting that the major efforts of research workers are devoted to such projects as testing hundreds of poisons to try to find one that will be more poisonous to malignant tissue than to healthy, nevertheless there are those who recognize the probable importance of this field of research. It is from such as these, striking out into radically new paths, that we hope for ultimately significant results that will help in the prevention of cancer.

One such daring research man is Lawrence LeShan of the Institute of Applied Biology in New York City. For the past 14 years Dr. LeShan has been studying what he calls the "emotional life histories" of adult cancer patients, looking for a common pattern that might be linked to the incidence of cancer. In April of 1965, when his study had been going on for 12 years, he was able to report on preliminary results to a conference on psychophysiological aspects of cancer held by the New York Academy of Sciences. At that time Dr. LeShan reported on 450 patients, all of whom had given extensive written personal histories on a well-designed test, and 150 of whom had been interviewed for an average of four hours each. Studying these histories, Dr. LeShan was able to find a remarkable similarity forming what he called a pattern of development and relationships that he found in 72 per cent of the

[83]

cancer patients, while the same pattern was found in only 10 per cent of the non-cancerous controls that he used. (Although he did not mention the possibility, it is not unlikely that cancer later developed or will develop in the 10 per cent of the controls who showed the same type of emotional pattern as that which was found dominant in cancer patients.)

Emotional Damage in Childhood

The first common element that Dr. LeShan stated as being dominant in emotional histories of cancer patients was that at some time during the first seven years of life, some kind of severe emotional experience damaged the ability of the child to relate to other people and to life itself. This could have been and often was a death in the family, such as the loss of one parent or of a brother or sister. In some cases it was simply the birth of a younger brother or sister and the loss of a great deal of parental attention and love which was shifted to the newborn. Whatever the specific cause, the child experienced a not uncommon reaction. Having loved someone fully and without qualification, the child experienced a deep pain and sense of loss at being deprived of that love, and came to the conclusion emotionally that it was safer not to love and not to risk the consequent pain of loss of the loved one.

This is a fairly common type of psychological development, leading in many children to an inner sense of guilt and a conviction of unworthiness to enjoy the love of others. Such children very quickly lose all conscious knowledge of why they have detached themselves emo-

[84]

tionally from the world around them and only feel that it is because of something missing in themselves, some lack of capacity for life, that they are not able to love people or enjoy living as others do.

Such a psychological deficiency rarely has any obvious signs. The child seems to be fairly well adjusted to the world around him. He does what he is supposed to do, he goes to school, he learns his lessons, he plays games with other children, and it is only by his lack of enthusiasm, perhaps by the inability to laugh, that an occasional perceptive adult may recognize there is something wrong. To most he seems perfectly normal, perhaps even better than others because he will tend to be unaggressive, having little that he really wants. He may also be very helpful to others, feeling more able to relate to the sick, the impoverished or the somehow enfeebled who by their very weakness represent less of a threat.

The net result in the young adult is frequently what is considered a "saintly" personality.

As we have seen before, this type of early personality development leads in turn to an utter devotion poured into a very narrow channel—a business, a husband or wife, perhaps a child. Here is Dr. LeShan's description of the situation:

"Some time in his development, usually in our cases in late adolescence or early adulthood, a situation arose that offered an opportunity for relating to others; a perceived change to end the deep loneliness he felt. This possibility seemed somehow 'safe'. Over a period of time, a period of slow and cautious experimentation,

[85]

he began to pour his energies into this channel. The feelings of isolation and 'lostness', the deep loneliness were greatly, but never completely, eased by this relationship. A tremendous amount of psychic and usually physical energy was poured into it. The cathexis (fixation of the libido or love drive onto an object) gave a meaning to life. For a period ranging from one year to over forty, they had a meaningful existence and a channel into which to pour their energy.

"Sometimes it was a job with a role for which they seemed particularly well adapted and which they enjoyed. Sometimes, as a spouse, a parent, or both, they found a way of life that brought them closer to satisfaction and relatedness than they had ever dreamed was possible. They still found it difficult to express or define their own wishes, but in the interest of their group or of the relationship, they could act very strongly.

"For a shorter or longer period, life continued on this plane. Then the blow fell. Circumstances brought an end to the relationship; their role was lost. Job retirement was forced on them, a spouse died, children grew up, became independent or no longer needed them. The immediate reaction varies. Some made desperate efforts to find substitute relationships. They tried to obtain new jobs, to make new friends, to find a new group, only to fail. Others were crushed by the blow. From a superficial view, all continued to 'adjust.' They continued to function and went about their daily business, but there was no more meaning and hope to their lives. Nothing gave them real satisfaction. It seemed to

[86]

them as though the thing they had expected and feared all their lives—utter isolation and rejection—was now their eternal doom. The only way out was to cease existing. 'Half in love with easeful death I cry' seemed to express their feelings. Although they feared death, they did not want to live.

"The early fantasy of something being basically wrong with them, something that made them unacceptable to others, returned in full force. Their energy level declined, because now there was no meaningful channel for its expression, and the decline was soon felt. The color and zest went out of life. *At some time from six months to 8 years after the crucial cathexis was lost, the first symptoms of cancer appeared in the cases we observed.*"

Dominated by Despair

Dr. LeShan found this same basic pattern repeated in 72 per cent of the 450 cancer cases whose emotional history he had painfully secured. What he considers the key factor is the ultimate quality of despair that dominates the person's life. And he defines it as hopelessness about ever achieving any real enjoyment or a real sense of meaning in life. Although the person tries and keeps on trying to establish meaningful relationships, it is always with an inner conviction that he is going to fail which in itself leads to failure.

One patient, when interviewed, said "I go on and I'm very efficient and I function very adequately, but this has nothing to do with the real me. Inside, none of this matters."

[87]

As a second described it, "It's as if all my life I've been climbing a very steep mountain. It's very hard work. Every now and then there are ledges I can rest on for a little bit, and maybe even enjoy myself a little, but I've got to keep climbing, and the mountain has no top."

A third described his life as being like a house with no insulation and with cracks in the walls. "The more heat you put in, the more heat leaks out. You can never get it warm."

And this type of personality, LeShan found, is overwhelmingly the type that contracts cancer. He carried his study further, however, examining his own and other statistics, particularly a study of the families of 200 breast cancer patients that was made in Copenhagen. This statistical study led LeShan to other significant conclusions. He found a statistical relationship, for example, between marital status and the incidence of cancer. The highest cancer rate was found among those who are widowed with the next highest rate among the divorced. The lowest rate is among single people, with the married in between. Reference to the census vital statistics for both the United States and the British Isles gave complete support to this thesis.

Finally LeShan asks the following significant question:

"Can psychological status of a patient affect the development of his tumor? If we accept a correlation between certain psychic states and neoplastic disease, what happens if the psychic states are modified? It is the author's strong *impression* that the psychotherapy

[88]

considerably slowed the development of the neoplasm, but no definitive proof can be given at the present time."

Regrettably, Dr. LeShan is in no sense a nutritionist. It apparently had never occurred to him to experiment with such elements as the vitamin-and enzyme-rich Gerson diets that significantly retarded and in some cases cured cases of cancer, or the large, therapeutic quantities of vitamin B and enzyme-rich desiccated liver and brewer's yeast that have been found in other experiments to act as a preventive of the development of cancer. Though we do not say it is so, it is at least possible that part of the effectiveness of these nutrients in combatting cancer may lie in their ability to improve the health of the nervous system and in this way improve and alter the emotional state.

There can be little doubt that there is a complicated and subtle interrelationship between the condition of health of the nerves and the way the mind operates. Which is the chicken and which the egg in the genesis of cancer is a question that no one has ever attempted to answer as yet.

Gardeners and Cancer

In *Prevention,* September, 1955, we published the idea of a doctor to the effect that gardeners suffered less cancer than nongardners.

It was a letter a doctor had sent to the editor of the *Medical Journal of Australia,* and which appeared in the January 22, 1955 issue of that publication. Here it is:

[89]

"Sir: It is my clinical impression that patients who are active gardeners have a much greater host resistance to internal carcinoma (cancer) than do nongardeners. Their survival period appears to be far greater in my experience. Whether this assumption is coincidental and false could be ascertained by practitioners working in city, suburban and country districts. May I, with respect, suggest this observation be made, and if established, submitted to the biochemists."

Yours, etc.,
Eric Goulston, M.D.
Sidney, December 20, 1954

I was terrifically excited about the item, and immediately got a letter off to Dr. Goulston, as follows:

Dear Dr. Goulston:

"I read your letter in the January 22, 1955 issue of the *Medical Journal of Australia* and I am wondering if you could give me more information about cancer and gardeners. We publish the magazine *Organic Gardening and Farming*, which represents Sir Albert Howard's idea of farming or gardening with nonchemical fertilizers.

Sincerely yours,
J.I. Rodale, Editor

Under date of April 4, 1955, I received the following reply from Dr. Goulston:

Dear Mr. Rodale:

"Thank you for your letter concerning cancer and gardeners. All I can say is that I have noticed over the years that there seems to be a greater host resistance against cancer in patients who are suffering from this disease and who delve in the garden, than is the case with complete non-gardeners. This may be due to some anti-carcinogenic agent ingested from soils or from plants. We are trying to investigate this problem bio-chemically but haven't got very far, so that at present, it is only a clinical impression.

"I would be very interested to learn if any similar work is being done in the States. Your idea of not farming with chemical fertilizers, would make an interesting study for a surgeon in your district to investigate and compare the incidence of cancer there as with other centres.

"I would like to hear from you again. I hope to visit the States next year, and if in Pennsylvania, I should like to make your acquaintance."

Dr. Goulston never visited me, nor did I know of any similar work done in this country. But I did have some gardening experience, and would like to express an opinion.

I would think that gardeners get more exercise in the open air, this oxygenating the body and causing it to function in a more efficient manner than that of a lethargic, nonactive person.

I have seen some cancer figures which showed that rural folk get less cancer than city people, which could be because they garden more.

It is a known fact that the earth contains electricity and magnetism. In fact it has been said that the world is one big magnet. We know also that the body is an

[91]

electrical power station, every cell being charged with electricity. Could it not be possible, therefore, that in placing the hands in the soil, an electric circuit between the body and earth is completed, and that some of the ground electricity gently begins to course through the body, invigorating the latter? In other words, if a person gardens every day, is he or she receiving a healthful daily electrical treatment?

But isn't it quite possible that the average gardener is a happier person than a non-gardener? I have known many gardeners in my time and my general impression is that they are more or less of a happy group.

The gardener has his little world, away from the world. While he gardens he forgets his troubles, which makes him happier while he is gardening than when he is not gardening.

The gardener sees the miracle of creation, the growth from the seed to the harvested plant. He sees flowers spring up as if by magic, and if he gardens a hundred years he will never cease to marvel, nor to enjoy his flowers, his vegetables or his fruit.

But your non-gardener will find a dozen reasons why not to garden. He will sit around brooding while his neighbor is reveling in his little plant world, weeds and all.

A survey should be made to check on cancer cases and whether they were gardeners. If there is a connection, then the Cancer Society could start a national publicity campaign to encourage people to go in for gardening.

Incidentally, in the July, 1960 *Organic Gardening*

and Farming, John H. Tobe, a famous nurseryman from Canada, wrote that a friend of his who had been on the Royal Canadian Mounted Police for 45 years had made thousands of arrests for crime, but not one of them was a nurseryman or an ardent gardener.

Pinning Down the Cancer Personality

Sometimes, when dealing with writings in the area of psychology, we have to stop and ask ourselves whether we really understand the terms describing personality that are used by psychologists. Their writings are not on the same level as medical literature. When a doctor refers to a tooth, a hangnail or a heart, we know exactly what he is talking about. Even if he uses an unfamiliar term such as, for example, *Escherichia coli,* all we have to do is go to the dictionary to learn that it is a type of bacteria with a precise shape that can be seen under the microscope and identified. But it is a very different matter when a psychologist refers to an "inhibited" or a "repressed" personality.

Just what do these words mean?

Even if we think we understand them, it is worthwhile checking on our understanding because so many people have written so much nonsense in the newspapers and magazines, using such terms loosely and very often without understanding themselves just what their terms mean. A lot of vulgar misconceptions have grown up, consequently. When we talk of an "inhibited" person, the first idea that leaps to mind is someone who does not permit himself to enjoy sex relations. But to a professional, inhibition may deal much more com-

[93]

monly and much more significantly with a person's inability to get angry when he is provoked, and a man may have a great relationship with his wife and still be inhibited as a psychologist sees him.

Thus it is appropriate to try to clarify for ourselves precisely which kind of people we are talking about when we quote the findings of various studies to the effect that those who develop cancer are characterized by repression and denial. Does this mean that these are people who won't spend the price of a new dress or suit? Are they abstemious in their eating habits or finicky about body odors or just what are they really like?

A descriptive paragraph would not tell us very much, since it would raise the same problem of just how to understand the words that are used. But there is a much clearer method that was used by Claus Bahne Bahnson and Marjorie Brooks Bahnson of the Jefferson Medical College in Philadelphia in a study they made. They conducted interviews with "24 patients, male and female, with different types and sites of cancer, from different walks of life, of different ages from 16 to 73, and living in different cities on the East Coast." Among other interview elements, these patients were asked long series of what are known as "forced-choice" interview questions. Such questions require that a statement be answered as either true or false, or in some cases that the one answering agrees or disagrees with the statement. Many such questions evoked such a random scattering of answers that they could be seen to have no particular significance. In some cases, however,

[94]

there was a remarkable degree of uniformity in the way the cancer patients answered a particular question.

All such questions were listed by Bahnson and Bahnson, with the result that we are able to get a much clearer picture of the cancer prone personality from the uniform attitudes of such personalities as reflected in their answers.

Here is one group of questions, and you will probably be as surprised as I was at how uniform the responses were and the specific type of personality they indicated.

	True	False
1. I was often sick to my stomach.	2	23
2. I could not keep my mind on any one thing.	3	22
3. I had periods of such great restlessness that I could not sit long in a chair.	4	21
4. My feelings were hurt easier than most people's.	3	22
5. A clear memory of my dreams often stayed with me for days.	4	21
6. My wife was not satisfied with my accomplishments in life.	4	21
7. At times I felt that I was going to crack up.	2	23
8. I can remember "playing sick" to get out of something.	1	24
9. I often had upsetting nightmares.	3	21
10. I felt hungry almost all the time.	2	23

[95]

11. When I went out, I usually preferred to go out by myself.	3	21
12. No one really understood me.	1	23
13. I often felt alone in the world.	3	22
14. Nothing turned out right for me.	3	22

Bahnson and Bahnson pointed out in reporting their study to the New York Academy of Sciences in 1965 that such uniform responses—far more uniform than were found in the responses of a control group of healthy people—could not be taken as representing the actual truth, but rather what these sick people wanted the truth to be.

". . . The cancer patients very definitely show a massive denial of all that can be embarrassing or is viewed as socially undesirable." In other words, these people were found to be socially conformist to such an exaggerated degree that even the mildest personality manifestation, such as having nightmares, that they thought other people might frown upon or consider queer, was immediately and unequivocally denied.

Not only were these cancer patients found to be unusually conformist, though, but it was also found that nearly uniformly their social attitudes depicted extreme conservatism and rectitude. These were the kind of people who would be pillars of whichever church they belonged to, dutiful hardworking employees, and more than a little stodgy—the kind of people who make others wonder what really goes on behind that mask of model behavior. Here are six typical questions which were answered with a startling uniformity.

	Agree	Disagree
1. Obedience and respect for authority are the most important virtues children should have.	22	2
2. Life is a serious business.	23	1
3. Honesty brings its own reward.	23	1
4. It is a wonderful feeling to sit surrounded by one's possessions.	18	6
5. Most people have a secret burden or cross to bear.	18	6
6. Most people are more nervous than appears on the surface.	21	3

Thus we began to get a picture of what it means in specific detail when earlier studies we have discussed have indicated that the cancer-prone temperament is repressed or inhibited or, what took us by surprise, extroverted. The repression is of behavior or even thoughts that it is felt would not be approved by one's parents in the first place or by society in general. The inhibition is no longer against sexual enjoyment which these days is hardly disapproved in the most conservative social circles, but rather against any type of behavior that might bring conflict with another person or people. And the extroversion is a technique of not feeling anti-social impulses by never examining oneself closely enough to be aware of them.

Another question used by Bahnson and Bahnson to define this special type of personality was: "When something makes you really angry which of the following are you likely to do?" The patient being questioned was presented with 15 different anger responses and asked whether he used each of these responses often, sometimes, or never. The grouping of the answers was highly revealing.

Only four of the group replied that they would strike back when angered, while nine asserted that they never strike back and 10 more were in between. Only 3 admitted to such a violent response as swearing, kicking or throwing things. While 23 conceded that getting angry could make them shake or tremble with rage, all but four asserted that they tried to keep their anger to themselves as long as possible. Nineteen asserted that they respond to anger by trying to think about more pleasant things, and 21 granted that they had a tendency to apologize even though they felt they were right.

Thus, through these questions, evoking specific situations, we get a very clear picture indeed of the kind of person who may be said to have a disposition toward contracting cancer. In a sense he might be said to have never grown up because, as an adult, he is still responding to the problems of his adult life in the same way he used to respond to the problems of family life as a child. When a father gets angry a child does not try to strike back and suppresses the anger with which he naturally reacts. And this type or response is necessary and wholesome for the child whose greatest need, after all, is for the authority of his parents to discipline him, to teach him how to behave, and to keep him out of trouble. Even though it evokes an instinctive resentment, authority to a child is the source of his security

[98]

and happiness. But as he grows older his personality should also be maturing, relying only on itself for authority and security, and able to express its mature needs and desires.

The adult who has never outgrown his childhood ways of reacting to a challenge is least likely to be aware of unhappiness and yet is most likely to be intrinsically a person who feels unexpressed and unfulfilled—an unhappy person.

Bahnson and Bahnson stated it like this:

"A study of the unstructured interviews with our cancer patients reveals that they all had experienced very close attachments to a parent or parent substitute early in life. Apparently, they had not been able to transcend genuinely the early dependency of their childhood, although in some cases they had been able to function adequately on the basis of reaction formation and over-compensation. However, in those cases, this compensatory way of dealing with the unsolved dependency needs had collapsed from one to two years prior to clinical onset of the malignancy. For most of the other patients unsatisfactory resolutions of early developmental problems had resulted in relationships during adult life which repeated the dependent childhood patterns. This solution, in turn, gave rise to severe conflicts with which the patients tried to cope by denying and repressing them, sometimes with success over long periods of time. This strategy resulted in a continual constriction of their life pattern and led them into more and more narrow, rigid, and barren terms of existence, until they regressed to living only in terms

[99]

of the most essential and narrow day-to-day routine. They then lived an emotionally frustrated, depleted, empty and barren life, with ever decreasing interpersonal stimulation and interaction, and with dwindling self-insight and self-communication. It was as if they then lived two lives: one formal, realistic, and common sense oriented, filling a social and family role with near perfection, but with another wounded and despairing self, existing independently and unrelated to the conscious and social self, thirsting for affection, warmth and personal creativity. Strikingly, from a clinical viewpoint, no communication whatever seemed to exist between these two 'selves.' A split and a role reversal, so to say, had taken place between primary and secondary process functioning. The regenerative drive seemed to have taken off on its own, having deprived the secondary process activities from the fuel which otherwise might have fired and intensified every day interpersonal life. Now it was closed off and went its own way.

"The theoretical points which have emerged from the clinical studies of our cancer patients thus are: (1) that underlying dependency and affectual needs remain infantile, (2) that serious frustrations result in narcissistic regression and re-organization, and (3) that due to repression and denial, available energy potentials under the reign of this self-propagating narcissism are retained on the primary process level, uncommunicable through the social self which atrophies and follows a bleak, repetitive routine.

[100]

CHAPTER XI

Cancer by the Can?

An unseemly fight broke out in the British House of Lords a few summers ago during a discussion over the chemicals in food, when Baroness Summerskill warned her fellow members that canned foods might cause cancer because of their metal content. She gave as evidence for her statement the history of a small colony of nuns in a remote part of Africa who lived mainly on canned foods, and among whom there was a high incidence of malignant diseases. The opposition countered with an expert opinion from the *London Times:* "One of the most foolish fallacies concerning 'tinned' foods is that they are liable to cause cancer."

The *British Medical Journal* (August 5, 1961) agreed that there is no real evidence that canned foods contain metals in harmful amounts. Perhaps this is true. We believe that if cancer comes from cans, it comes less from what is in canned foods, than what is

[101]

not in them. The greatest damage done by a diet of processed foods is the nutrition it lacks. Your body needs nutrition to protect itself from cancer. Technical books on food processing make it very clear that canned foods are sadly lacking in it.

Enzymes Destroyed

In *The Technology of Food Preservation* by Norman W. Desrosier, Ph.D., Professor of Food Technology at Purdue University, the nutrition-damaging effects involved in canning are outlined in detail. Consider the inactivation of enzymes. Enzymes must be stopped in their tracks in any type of food preservation, since they bring food to the point of maturity, and will continue past that point to overripeness and deterioration, if they are not inactivated. In other methods of preserving food (freezing and dehydration) serious attention is paid to averting complete destruction of enzymes, but not in canning. Some experts say that enzymes are permanently destroyed by heat at any point above 122 degrees fahrenheit. When food is prepared for canning it is heated to well above 122 degrees, and heated again when the housewife prepares it for the table. A diet consisting exclusively of canned food would have to be utterly deficient in enzymes.

Every cell of every tissue needs enzymes to trigger the thousands of chemical processes that are going on inside you as you read this. Each part of the body manufactures some of the enzymes that function there —the heart muscle makes its own and so do the leg muscles, the muscles in the eye, etc. If an enzyme neces-

[102]

sary for some step in the metabolic process happens to be missing, illness or death will probably result.

The foods we eat contain enzymes and can supplement the human enzyme supply, fill in, as it were, when the body is short of its own enzymes. The enzymes we get in raw foods are called exogenous enzymes. The more you get of these, the less endogenous enzymes (those produced by your body) you need. Researchers find the body's response to the enzymes in food so gratifying that they have begun using them therapeutically. Papain, extracted from the papaya, for example, is used to treat bedsores, skin allergies, hemmorhoids and heart disease.

Raw food contains a great store of natural enzymes; heat-processed foods contain none at all. Enzymes are essential to proper release of other nutrients in the foods we eat. A steady diet of enzyme-poor canned foods will drastically reduce the amount of necessary vitamins and minerals available to the body.

Desrosier's book makes it clear that protein is denatured by the high heat used in the canning process. The natural configuration of the protein molecule is lost. It is known that animals thrive less well on highly heated protein than on slightly heated protein.

An inefficient protein supply in the system can lead to a list of diseases that is almost endless. The antibodies the blood manufactures to fight disease are protein; so a lack of protein leaves the door open to all kinds of infections and viruses. If cancer is a virus, a protein-deficient system is easy prey for cancer. Protein also protects the liver against poisonous chemicals.

[103]

Finally, we know that vitamins and minerals cannot be used by the body unless the proper hormones and enzymes are there to combine with them. Hormones and enzymes are made of protein.

Vitamins Adversely Affected

Vitamin losses in canned foods are commonly acknowledged in science, and pretty familiar even to the lay public. Just about all of the B vitamins are affected adversely. In the *American Journal of Surgery* (August, 1942) Hayes Martin, M.D., suggested that many of the symptoms people complain about in the region of their mouths, tongues, lips, gums (ulcers, boils or patches of inflammation, white spots that have appeared on the gums or insides of the cheeks, etc.) are what they term "precancerous." This does not mean that cancer is caused by these disorders. It means that a body condition that produces such disorders in the mouth may later produce cancer. A study of 300 patients at Memorial Hospital in New York showed that those suffering from mouth disorders, ranging all the way from the slightest irritation to advanced cancer of the mouth, were short on vitamin B. They found, too, that in general, other symptoms of B deficiency accompanied the mouth symptoms in these patients.

Dr. H. F. Kraybill, Ph.D., of the National Cancer Institute, wrote in *Clinical Pharmacology and Therapeutics* (January-February, 1963): "Yeast, (rich in B vitamins) is particularly effective for the prevention of liver cancer since the level of 15 per cent of it is almost completely protective and any high-quality pro-

[104]

tein diet and B vitamins, especially B₂, are defensive mechanisms in the inhibiting formations of such neoplasms." Dr. Kraybill went on to say, "Consideration of food intake in carcinogenesis is not restricted to nutrition *per se* but must also include additives, contaminants, or processing degradation products which may play a more important role in tumor induction."

Vitamin C

Vitamin C is destroyed by heating at low temperatures for long periods of time. If oxygen is present the destruction is even swifter. Vitamin C has achieved a reputation for being the most destructible vitamin. Canned foods, heated in processing, and heated again before being served, are almost sure to have lost a minimum of two-thirds of their original vitamin C value.

In the *Archives of Pediatrics* (October, 1954) W. J. McCormick, M.D., suggested that one solution to our cancer problem might be a change in diet and environment that would bring us all ample supplies of vitamin C. Several researchers have found that there is a pronounced C deficiency in the blood of cancer patients, compared to that of healthy persons. It has been found that guinea pigs suffering from scurvy (the disease of vitamin C deficiency), and given just enough vitamin C to keep alive, are far more susceptible to cancer and get it sooner than healthy guinea pigs.

We know that the cement holding cells together (collagen) can be manufactured only if vitamin C is present in ample quantity. This cement becomes watery in an individual suffering from scurvy. The protein contained normally in this cement disappears into the blood. In cancer patients, tests show an increase of this particular protein in the blood. When vitamin C is given, almost immediately the intracellular cement begins to form in its normal consistency.

It becomes obvious from even these few references, that anyone eating a highly processed diet runs a much greater risk of contracting cancer, aside from any contaminants in the cans, than the individual who eats fresh foods frequently. The argument in the House of Lords concentrated on a rather superficial aspect of canned foods and their relationship to cancer. Cancer may or may not result from stray metals in canned foods. Few, if any, pathologists would argue against the possibility that cancer and a diet almost exclusively made up of canned foods are dangerously compatible.

Of course our advice is to include as many fresh, unprocessed foods in your diet as possible. For those people who, for one reason or another, find their diet overloaded with processed foods, the best security and protection is a regular schedule of natural vitamins, particularly those rich in the B complex such as brewer's yeast, desiccated liver and wheat germ. Rose hips and acerola will fill in for vitamin C, and the unsaturated fats are plentiful in vegetable oils such as safflower oil, olive oil and sunflower seed oil.

Nutritional deficiency in canned foods is not the only road that can lead to cancer, but it is certainly a well-traveled one that should be considered in a program of disease avoidance.

[106]

Part Two:

THE ACCEPTED
TREATMENTS

CHAPTER XII

Treating Cancer, prepared by the U.S. Public Health Service

A booklet prepared and published by:

U.S. Department of Health, Education, and Welfare
Public Health Service

Diagnosing Cancer

Patients with cancer that is diagnosed when it is still localized, or restricted to a limited area, have the best chance for cure. Because symptoms do not usually become obvious to a patient until the disease is well under way, regular examinations, particularly for people over 40, play an important role in cancer detection.

The doctor may use a variety of techniques, but the only sure way he can determine whether or not a growth is cancer is to perform a biopsy. This is usually a minor surgical procedure which involves removing some of the suspicious tissue and examining it under a microscope.

A medical specialist known as a pathologist can

recognize characteristic malignant, or cancerous cells if they are present in the specimen. Malignant cells are usually irregular in size and shape and have large nuclei and abnormal chromosomes. Malignant tissue generally has a disorganized appearance and sometimes shows areas of cell destruction.

Some tumors are benign, or non-cancerous. Under the microscope, benign tumor tissue usually appears orderly, and the individual cells appear similar.

The major difference between malignant and benign tumors is the ability of malignant cells to spread to areas beyond the original tumor. A malignant tumor may spread by direct invasion of the surrounding tissues, or cancer cells may break off and spread through the blood or lymph systems, a process known as metastasis. Benign tumors, often enclosed in a capsule, do not spread.

In some cases it may be necessary for the surgeon to perform an "exploratory" operation. A biopsy specimen taken during an exploratory operation can be examined at once. If the specimen shows that cancer is present, the necessary surgery can be performed while the patient is still on the operating table, thus sparing him another major operation.

Exfoliative cytology, the examination of cells shed from the surface of tissues into body cavities, is one of the most useful aids to diagnosis, particularly in screening large or high risk population groups.

The "Pap" test, for example, permits detection of cancer of the uterine cervix by examination of cells shed from the uterus. As a result of the wide-spread use of this test, deaths from cancer of the uterus have been substantially reduced.

Cells shed from the stomach, esophagus, lung, colon, and bladder have also been examined. These techniques are particularly useful in cases where the presence of cancer is suspected.

X-rays are an important detection tool, especially for cancer of the lung and parts of the digestive tract. X-ray examination of the breast by a procedure known as mammography is an experimental technique that may be useful in screening large groups of women for breast cancer. Studies have shown that mammography can detect some breast tumors before they can be felt.

The doctor can also detect tumors deep within the body by using special instruments that are essentially hollow, lighted tubes. For example, a bronchoscope enables him to study parts of the lung, and a sigmoidoscope helps him study parts of the lower digestive tract.

The patient's physician is in the best position to decide what treatment is best for a particular patient since he has the most complete information about the case. The factors influencing the kind of treatment are the type, extent, and location of cancer, and the age and general health of the patient.

Surgery

The aim of treatment is complete removal of the tumor, including surrounding tissues into which the cancer may have extended. Surgical removal of a tumor usually causes no change in the patient's funda-

[111]

mental body processes, although in some cases adjustments may have to be made. For example, if the larynx or "voice box" is removed, the patient will have to learn a new way to talk. If the rectum is removed, a temporary or permanent opening known as a colostomy may be made in the abdominal wall.

Surgery usually does not change the general appearance of the patient. If scars are left, plastic surgery is often helpful. In recent years, a large number of new artificial materials have been developed that help restore the patient's appearance.

In order to prevent distant metastases, surgeons often remove lymph nodes near the tumor if there is a suspicion that cancer has spread to these structures. Once metastasis to distant organs has occurred, chances for cure are greatly lessened.

Another example of cancer surgery is the removal of hormone sources, such as the ovaries, adrenal glands, or the pituitary gland, which influence the growth of certain organs and tumors derived from these organs. Thus, a surgeon might remove ovaries from a woman with breast cancer in an effort to check its growth.

If the patient is suffering from incurable cancer, the surgeon is sometimes able to perform an operation that will relieve pain. Such an operation may involve severing nerves either at the place where the cancer started, or to which it has spread.

Preventive surgery is sometimes performed to remove certain types of polyps and moles which are considered to be precancerous conditions.

The patient who undergoes surgery today has a

better chance for cure than ever before in history. The development of improved operating procedures and increased knowledge of principles of pre- and post-operative care have contributed to the greater safety and effectiveness of surgery.

Very complex, and increasingly extensive, or "radical" operations of the internal organs and the head and neck can now be performed. Availability of improved anesthetic techniques, antibiotics to control infection, blood transfusions, and muscle relaxing drugs have made these operations possible.

Efforts to bring the patient to the best possible state of health before and after an operation also contribute to the effectiveness of modern surgery. For some time after an operation, the patient is closely observed by hospital personnel trained to recognize and treat possible complications.

The surgical patient is advised to walk and exercise soon after his operation, and to help care for himself. Encouragement and medical care after he leaves the hospital are essential for complete recovery.

Research and Surgery

Scientists are conducting research to increase chances for cure by surgery. Some of their studies are aimed at explaining the reasons for failure of surgery to cure some cancer.

Some scientists think that at the time of surgery, cancer cells may contaminate the wound or be released to migrate through the body, causing tumors to recur months after apparently successful surgery. By combin-

[113]

ing surgery with drug or radiation treatment, they are trying to alter the cells of the tumor so that if the cells spread during or soon after the operation, they will be incapable of growing at a new site.

Other investigators are developing new surgical techniques and tools. The laser, an optical instrument that emits a narrow beam of intense light, has been found to destroy certain experimental tumors in laboratory animals. Experimental tumors have also been destroyed by freezing with liquid nitrogen, a technique known as cryosurgery. Another new technique, known as chemosurgery, involves the use of a chemical agent or drugs that destroy skin cancer. These techniques are not meant to replace surgery, but they may someday help surgeons bring certain forms of cancer under control.

Radiation

Radiation is another type of definitive and, in some cases, curative cancer treatment. It has been in use for more than 60 years, and today some form of radiation is used in treating about 6 out of every 10 cancer patients.

Radiation may be of several types. X-rays, electromagnetic waves similiar to light and heat waves, are produced in a machine and are an important form of artificial radiation. In the X-ray machine, fast-moving electrons strike a metal target, and the energy of their motion is converted in part to X-rays. By varying the voltage in the X-ray vacuum tube, X-rays of high or low energy may be produced.

Certain elements, known as radioactive isotopes,

spontaneously emit radiation. Radium and uranium are well-known radioisotopes that occur in nature, but they are very rare. Other elements can be made radioactive by bombarding them with high velocity atomic particles. These particles are produced in atom-smashing devices such as the nuclear reactor, the cyclotron, and the Van de Graaf accelerator.

Soon after radiation was discovered, late in the 19th century, scientists found that it sometimes damaged body tissues. Later studies showed that an amount of radiation which had a tolerated effect on normal tissue caused considerable damage to cancer tissue and sometimes completely destroyed the cancer.

To cure cancer, a radiation dose must be large enough to destroy cancer cells, but not so great as to damage seriously normal tissue surrounding or overlying the cancer. Some types of cancer, including cancer of the gastrointestinal tract and associated organs, are not usually destroyed by radiation that is within a dose range safe to surrounding normal tissues and therefore are considered resistant to radiation. Cancer of most other sites may be treated by radiation.

Radiation is very effective against certain cancers arising from the lymphatic and blood-forming systems, including Hodgkin's disease, lymphosarcoma, and some forms of leukemia. It is also useful in combination with surgery or drugs in treating Ewing's tumor, a kind of bone tumor; Wilms' tumor, a cancer of the kidney in children; and retinoblastoma, a childhood cancer of the eye.

Early, localized Hodgkin's disease is best treated by

[115]

large doses of X-rays. In fact, localized Hodgkin's disease can be completely controlled in more than 50 per cent of the patients for periods exceeding 15 years.

A combination of radiation with drug treatment has many uses. For example, the drug actinomycin D appears to enhance the effect of radiation in treating Wilms' tumor. Radiation is sometimes used to shrink the size of a tumor before surgery or to help prevent metastasis at the time of surgery.

The kind of tumor and its location determine the amount and kind of X-ray treatment given. High energy X-rays, which penetrate deeply into the body, are used to treat cancer of the internal organs, while low energy X-rays may be used to treat superficial cancers of the mouth and skin.

In recent years, supervoltage on multimillion volt X-ray machines have been developed. Their advantage is that their rays are more penetrating, scatter less radiation through the body, and irradiate a smaller zone of normal tissue than low voltage machines.

Radioactive isotopes are used to treat many forms of cancer, including cancer of the mouth, larynx or esophagus, prostate, uterine cervix, and body of the uterus. Radium, cobalt-60, and other radioisotopes may be beamed to the body through the use of a pack, or "bomb." In this procedure, a small amount of radioactive material is enclosed in a shielded unit and the beams are directed to the patient through a shutter. The "bomb" can be rotated around the patient so that cancer tissue receives a maximum dose of radiation while healthy tissue receives a minimum; this is more

[116]

practical than rotating the patient for the same purpose.

The advantages of the cobalt-60 bomb have made it a popular source of radiation therapy, especially in treating deep seated cancer. Use of this machine makes possible administration of large doses of radiation to a greater depth with less harmful side effects than conventional low energy X-rays. In addition, cobalt-60 is one of the cheapest radioisotopes available.

In some cases radioisotopes may be placed directly on or in the body. As solids they may be placed on the skin, inserted in body cavities, or implanted in tissues. Devices such as needles, plaques, seeds, wires, wax molds, and capsules have been created to place the radiation source as close as possible to the cancer. For example, radium needles may be implanted to treat cancer of the mouth, and radium enclosed in a capsule may be inserted into the uterine cavity. Radioisotopes in liquid form may be injected into cavities or tissues, or mingled with body fluids for transport to interior parts of the body. Sometimes radioactive gold or phosphorus may be injected into the area of a prostate tumor.

Radioactive Tracers

Radioisotopes that tend to concentrate in a particular body tissue are useful in both diagnosis and treatment of cancer. Normal thyroid tissue, for example, collects most of the body's iodine to use in the manufacture of thyroid hormone. Sometimes thyroid cancer cells that have spread to other parts of the body con-

[117]

tinue to collect iodine, and will take up radioactive iodine. By first giving the patient with thyroid cancer a "tracer dose" of radioactive iodine, and then passing a counter over the patient's body, a doctor can tell whether widespread iodine-collecting deposits of cancer cells are present. The next step is usually surgical removal of the thyroid gland, if this has not been done already. This measure is followed by giving the patient hormones to stimulate activity in the thyroid tissue that has spread to other parts of the body. The doctor then has the patient drink an "atomic cocktail" of radioactive iodine, which destroys those cancer tissues that pick up a sufficient amount of it. Such a procedure sometimes controls thyroid cancer for years. Similarly, radioactive phosphorus collects in bone and its dividing cells and is used in treating certain types of cancer of the blood and bone.

Research in Radiation Therapy

Scientists are conducting research on ways of increasing the effectiveness of radiation treatment. In some hospitals, cancer patients have been irradiated in chambers containing pressurized oxygen following tests which indicate a high concentration of oxygen makes cancer more vulnerable to radiation.

An area of great current interest is the potential use of neutrons, another form of radiation, in patient treatment. Neutrons appear to have the capacity to partially overcome the resistance of cancer cells to conventional types of radiation (X-rays, cobalt or radium gamma rays).

[118]

Another approach is the use of chemicals to increase the radiosensitivity of cancer cells or to protect normal tissues from radiation damage. Other investigations have centered on methods of giving higher doses of radiation without increasing the side effects. Total body irradiation given in multiple small doses has, in some patients, produced complete disappearance of tumors with minimal effect on normal tissues. Diseases shown to be responsive to this type of treatment to date include widespread lymphomas such as lymphosarcoma and chronic lymphocytic leukemia.

Recently, it has been found possible to extend the usefulness of radiation therapy in Hodgkin's disease to cases with involvement of multiple lymph node areas. By the use of carefully designed treatment schedules, large doses of radiation have been delivered to the many areas known to contain tumor. This has resulted in complete remissions in a majority of patients and the side effects of such extensive irradiation have been tolerated satisfactorily. Whether this technique will produce cures in these more advanced cases, as can be accomplished with localized Hodgkin's disease, will require a longer period of evaluation than is available at present.

Another technique involves transplanting bone marrow to cancer patients whose bone marrow has been severely depressed by large doses of radiation. Scientists are experimenting with the replacement of damaged marrow with some removed from the patient before treatment and stored at low temperatures, or with marrow donated by close relatives.

[119]

These research efforts hold considerable promise for improving the effectiveness of radiotherapy in the management of cancer. It may be hopefully anticipated that such research will lead to an increasingly significant role of radiation.

Chemotherapy

Localized cancer often can be removed by surgery or destroyed by radiation. But these methods can rarely cure cancers that have spread, nor can they cure cancers of the blood or blood-forming tissues, such as leukemia, which are widespread from the beginning. Most of the 300,000 cancer deaths yearly in the United States are due to inability of surgery or radiation to cure widespread disease.

Scientists have felt for many years that the best way to treat such cancers would be with drugs, or chemicals, that would destroy cancer cells and yet not harm normal, healthy tissue. But not until the mid-1940's was there any evidence that drugs would be useful in treating cancer.

Some two dozen drugs have now been developed that are temporarily effective in the treatment of cancer. In a few cases they can produce cures; in most cases they temporarily stop the growth of certain cancers, relieve pain, and allow the patient to live a longer, more comfortable life.

In most cases, the drugs eventually lose their effect against cancer, for reasons that are not entirely known. One explanation may be that the cancer cells multiply more rapidly than the drugs can kill them. The admin-

[120]

istration of drugs is limited by the side effects that often appear, such as impaired production of blood cells, temporary loss of hair, and nausea, vomiting, and diarrhea.

Alkylating Agents

Chemical agents that have been effective in cancer therapy are of several types. One group is known as alkylating agents. Because their effect on tissue mimics radiation, they are sometimes called radiomimetic agents. Like radiation, these drugs also damage normal cells and consequently have limited use.

Nitrogen mustard and other chemicals related to the wartime "poison gases" are alkylating agents that have produced temporary relief in patients with certain cancers of the lymphatic and blood-forming tissues, such as Hodgkin's disease, lymphosarcoma, and chronic leukemia. The nitrogen mustards are also useful in treating lung and breast cancer.

Cyclophosphamide has produced similar effects against blood cancers, multiple myeloma, and breast and ovarian cancers. Other alkylating agents are chlorambucil (thio-TEPA, TEM), and busulfan (Myleran).

Metabolic Antagonists

Another group of chemotherapeutic agents are the metabolic antagonists, or antimetabolites. These agents are designed to starve cancer cells by interfering with vital life processes. They are "counterfeit building blocks," materials that closely resemble those needed by the cancer cell in its development. They "fool" the cell into using them with the result that the

[121]

cell's processes are faulty and its activity is blocked. As with all chemotherapeutic agents, treatment of cancer with antimetabolites is limited. Antimetabolites may also damage normal cells.

Perhaps the most widely used of the metabolic antagonists are the folic acid antagonists which are related to the vitamin, folic acid. Methotrexate (amethopterin), chief among these antagonists, has been particularly useful for the treatment of acute leukemia in children.

Encouraging success has been observed in the use of methotrexate in treating choriocarcinoma, a rare kind of cancer that follows pregnancy. Methotrexate treatment resulted in long-term remissions approaching cures in approximately 50 per cent of patients with widespread disease. Even better survival results were produced by the sequential use of methotrexate and an antibiotic, actinomycin D. In both localized and widespread disease, methotrexate has produced complete remissions without the need for surgical removal of the uterus, allowing the patient to retain child-bearing capacity.

The counterfeit purines are another group of metabolic antagonists. Chief among these is 6-mercaptopurine, which has been used to treat acute leukemia in children and chronic and acute leukemia in adults.

Another class of antimetabolites is the fluorinated pyrimidines. Dramatic, though temporary, results have been obtained by physicians using 5-FU and its derivative, 5-FUDR, to treat patients with a wide variety of tumors.

[122]

Hormones

Some cancers of the breast, prostate, and uterus occur in tissues influenced by hormones. Some of these cancers tend to appear at a time of life when hormonal activity in the body has changed; after menopause, for example.

Treatment with hormones may affect these cancers through changing the hormonal environment. For example, male hormones, or androgens, are sometimes effective in treating young women with advanced breast cancer. Women who have breast cancer that cannot be treated by surgery, and who are past the menopause, have responded favorably to treatment with female hormones, or estrogens.

Other hormonal agents have shown value in treating some cancers of the blood-forming organs. Improvement in adults as well as in children with acute leukemia has been produced by prednisone or predniosolene, derivatives of the adrenal hormone, cortisone. Progesterone, a hormone that influences the lining of the uterus (the endometrium) is used to treat endometrial cancer.

Other Anticancer Drugs

The drugs vincristine and vinblastine are compounds derived from the common periwinkle plant. Vincristine is one of the most important drugs used to treat acute leukemia, Hodgkin's disease and breast cancer, and is also useful against Wilms' tumor and rhabdomyosarcoma. A compound, o,p'-DDD, closely related to the

[123]

insecticide DDT, is the most effective agent against cancer of the adrenal glands. Actinomycin D, an antibiotic, is used in combination with radiation to treat Wilms' tumor, and is also useful in treating testicular cancer, rhabdomyosarcoma, and choriocarcinoma.

Drugs Used To Treat Cancer

alkylating agents	busulfan (Myleran) chlorambucil cyclophosphamide nitrogen mustard phenylalanine mustard (Melphalan) Thio-TEPA Triethylene melamine (TEM)
antimetabolites	methotrexate (amethopterin) 5-fluorouracil (5-FU) 6-mercaptopurine
hormonal agents adrenal cortical compounds	cortisone hydrocortisone prednisolone prednisone
androgens (male sex hormones)	fluoxymesterone testosterone propionate
estrogens (female sex hormones)	diethylstilbestrol ethinyl estradiol
other	progesterone ACTH
miscellaneous	actinomycin D methyl-GAG methyl hydrazine o,p'-DDD vinblastine vincristine

[124]

Type of Cancer	*Drugs Used*
acute lymphocytic leukemia	methotrexate, 6-mercapto-purine, cyclophosphamide, adrenal cortical compounds, ACTH, vincristine
acute granulocytic leukemia	6-mercaptopurine, methyl-GAG
chronic lymphocytic leukemia	busulfan, 6-mercaptopurine
Hodgkin's disease	chlorambucil, cyclophospha-mide, nitrogen mustard, Thio-TEPA, TEM, vinblastine, vincristine, methyl hydrazine
lymphosarcoma	chlorambucil, clyclophosph-amide, nitrogen mustard, Thio-TEPA, TEM, adrenal cortical compounds, vincris-tine, vinblastine
multiple myeloma	cyclophosphamide, phenyla-lanine mustard
choriocarcinoma	methotrexate, 6-mercaptopur-ine, actinomycin D, vinblastine
breast cancer	chlorambucil, cyclophospha-mide, nitrogen mustard, Thio-TEPA, TEM, methotrexate, 5-FU, male sex hormones, female sex hormones, adrenal cortical compounds, vinblastine
ovarian cancer	chlorambucil, cyclophospha-mide, nitrogen mustard, Thio-TEPA, TEM, vinblastine
testicular cancer	chlorambucil, methotrexate, actinomycin D
endometrial cancer	progesterone
Wilm's tumor	actinomycin D, vincristine
retinoblastoma	Thio-TEPA, TEM
lung cancer	nitrogen mustard, cyclophos-phamide, 5-FU
colon cancer	5-FU
stomach cancer	5-FU
adrenal cancer	o,p'-DDD
rhabdomyosarcoma	actinomycin D, vincristine

Cancer Chemotherapy Research

A national cooperative chemotherapy program sponsored by the National Cancer Institute is being conducted to further the search for drugs to cure cancer. It involves many research laboratories in the Government, in universities and medical schools, and in the pharmaceutical industry.

Each year, approximately 17,000 materials are tested. These materials are chemicals, plant extracts, antibiotics, and newly synthesized compounds related to known drugs. They are tested for anticancer activity against certain rat and mouse tumors that have been shown to be predictive of antitumor activity in man. Those that appear active are then tested in larger animals for evidence of toxicity. About one out of every 1,000 of these chemicals is considered promising and safe enough to be studied in patients. This is being done in a number of hospitals throughout the country.

These clinical studies are helping to determine the most effective methods of administering drugs to achieve the main goal of chemotherapy research—the destruction of all cancer cells with minimum harm to normal cells. An important recent advance toward this goal has been use of intensive treatment of acute leukemia with combinations of drugs.

Several procedures have been devised for minimizing the toxicity of anticancer drugs. One method is introduction of drugs directly into the blood in the cancer-affected area by a process known as regional perfusion. A drip-in or infusion pump may be used to

[126]

deliver a measured amount of the drug to the cancer site.

Among drug developments are efforts to find some that will pass from the general circulation to the central nervous system and brain where, for example, leukemic cells may "hide out." Most of the drugs now in use do not pass the "blood-brain barrier." A new agent, BCNU, is one that can pass this barrier and it has been found highly effective against mouse leukemia. Its delayed harmful effects in man restrict its use at present.

Some anticancer drugs interfere with the production of essential blood elements, leaving the patient vulnerable to complicating infections and hemorrhages. Prevention and treatment of these complications has been a major factor in prolonging the lives of leukemic children. To control hemorrhage, patients can be given transfusions of platelets, the blood element that induces clotting. At present, 32 medical centers have joined a National Cancer Institute-sponsored program of platelet transfusion therapy.

To control infections, antibiotics are given and methods for replacing infection-fighting white cells are being developed. Ways of preventing infection are also being studied. Some patients are given anticancer drugs while isolated in a germfree environment—a plastic enclosed chamber—to reduce the possibility of infection.

Scientists are trying to find out if they can use the body's natural defense—its immunological system—to control cancer. This system consists of specialized

[127]

groups of cells that recognize and reject some foreign substances, or antigens. They produce specific counter-substances called antibodies that react with and inactivate the antigens.

Although cancer tissue differs from normal tissue, no tumor antigen has yet been isolated from a human tumor. Therefore, the possibility of using a vaccine made of cancer cells to stimulate production of antibodies against the cancer is still far in the future.

Perhaps this research will someday lead to an immunological approach to cancer treatment. But until much more work is done in this area, surgery, radiation, and chemotherapy remain the only methods of treating cancer.

Part Three:

TREATMENTS NOT OFFICIALLY ACCEPTED

CHAPTER XIII

Enzyme Treatment and the Double Standard

In the Government's continuing search for a cure for cancer, two huge federal agencies, the Food and Drug Administration (FDA) and the National Cancer Institute (NCI), play dominant, and even commanding roles. Now, strong criticism of their performance has been voiced on the floor of the United States Senate by Edward V. Long (Democrat-Missouri). Drawing upon the findings of an intensive six-month study by his medical adviser, Dr. Miles H. Robinson of Potomac, Maryland, Senator Long has posed many questions that touch on the relation of government-sponsored research to the individual doctor, and eventually to the cancer patient himself.

The Robinson study fundamentally attacks what its author calls "the FDA's double standard" in approving

[131]

the testing of anti-cancer drugs. The criticism is that the FDA lets the NCI get away with numerous procedures that it would not allow the private, non-government-financed researcher to follow.

The particular focus of Dr. Robinson's study is the case of Dr. Franklin L. Shively of Dayton, Ohio, who has been attempting to use injections of enzymes in the treatment of cancer. Enzymes are protein substances that trigger nearly all of the body's chemical processes. The enzymes that Dr. Shively was injecting into his hospitalized patients are all found in the human body, Dr. Robinson noted in his study.

Enzyme Studies Needed

The use of enzymes has been urged by several outstanding cancer researchers in Europe, but the idea has not yet taken hold among the vast majority of researchers. As Dr. Robinson explained in an interview, the most prevalent theory about the cancer cell was that it was a rapid multiplier, with too great an enzyme activity, and reproduced itself in a wild, uncontrolled, explosive growth. "Now there is the feeling that cancer cells are like juvenile delinquents in that they have escaped from the normal control of the body and are driven to inconsiderate growth—but that their pattern of enzyme activity is usually depressed when compared to normal cells," Dr. Robinson said.

"Thus, one theoretical object of giving extra enzymes to cancer patients is to try to raise the low enzyme activity of cancerous cells," he added.

Dr. Shively treated 193 patients with various en-

[132]

zymes over a period of some 12 years. While Dr. Robinson emphasized that no one was making any definite claims, he pointed out that there had been some beneficial results. The FDA, he charged, has been blocking further research by Dr. Shively by imposing numerous bureaucratic regulations, while, Dr. Robinson feels, not requiring similar procedures from NCI scientists and doctors.

The NCI is still, according to Dr. Robinson, dominated by the longstanding medical belief that toxic chemicals, such as mustard gas derivatives, among others, offer the best approach to chemical cures for cancer. The NCI has tested some 170,000 possible anti-cancer chemicals at a cost of $500 million without yet coming up with anything really definitive.

The toxic chemical approach to cancer cure stems largely from the idea that the cancer cells, since they are a wild outgrowth, might be destroyed by the chemical. The patient obviously will suffer toxic effects, but the idea is that somehow he will not quite succumb to it, but that the cancer cells will. Dr. Robinson attacks this concept in his study, favoring the Shively idea of the use of the body's own chemicals, enzymes, in combating tumors.

A major part of the Robinson study condemns what it calls the lax standards of NCI testing, and there are strong statements to the effect that the "little men"— the Dr. Shivelys, who do not have institutional prestige—are much more severely regulated than is the NCI. Dr. Robinson also accuses the FDA of considerable footdragging in attending to Dr. Shively's requests for clearance for further research. FDA procedures requires a researcher to submit detailed statements of what he proposes to do and how. Dr. Robinson charges the FDA with a seven-month delay in handling Dr. Shively's applications. He had been ordered to halt his treatments, pending a further FDA review. He complied.

Lax Procedures at NCI

Much more serious, Dr. Robinson condemns NCI testing procedures as having harmed patients and as, in many cases, being conducted without the knowledge of the sick people themselves. He cites a number of cases, some from the NCI's own reports, of where there was toxic effect from chemical cancer treatment. But Dr. Robinson is quick to note that it is not possible to determine whether people who are desperately ill with cancer die eventually from that disease or from the particular chemical treatment. Nevertheless, he leaves the definite impression that NCI chemical tests have caused needless and considerable suffering.

He also hammers hard at the point that the great medical bureaucracies at the FDA and NCI treat each other with a circumspection that does not extend to the individual medical researcher who labors in his own laboratory unfinanced by any government grant. Running all through Dr. Robinson's discussion of the relation between big government medical research and the lone researcher is the implication that the bureaucrats are too concerned with politics, prestige, and career advancement. This feeling is also apparent when he speaks with admiration approaching a kind of awe of the triumphs that lonely men working late on their own have achieved in the past. But, as Dr. Robinson would most certainly if ruefully have to admit, the trend nowadays is toward research by committee, and the big scientists of this era may well be men more gifted in administration and political skills than in the traditional laboratory techniques.

Dr. Robinson's study emphasizes strongly his belief in the ingrained dislike of the medical establishment—that is, the big government medical agencies, major medical schools, and prestige hospitals—for new, unorthodox treatment of a given disease. In his impassioned defense of Dr. Shively, Dr. Robinson is almost pleading with the establishment to reverse its traditional bent and give the Shively treatment a complete and unprejudiced examination. Dr. Robinson notes that the NCI, having all but exhausted chemicals in its search for a cancer treatment, will now begin moving slowly into the enzyme field. The idea of spending half a billion dollars in a vast attempt to come up with some kind of chemical treatment has been seen by many as an indication of desperation on the part of the government.

The desperation is justified, given the appalling nature and numbers of the cancer problem, but what Dr. Robinson now hopes is that the FDA and the NCI will give enzymes and Dr. Shively a chance. It is noted that all the chemical testing heretofore by NCI has produced only a few moderately effective treatments

[135]

in a few kinds of cancer—nothing even approaching a cure.

As both Senator Long and Dr. Robinson note, all clinical research on drugs is subject to the absolute control of the FDA. Yet the FDA has not the staff to have great expertise in the specialized area of cancer, and, therefore, must rely on the judgment of NCI scientists. Thus, there is the odd situation of FDA having to rely on NCI in the search for a chemical treatment, and yet it must also regulate NCI's procedures where drug testing on patients is concerned. The result, according to the Robinson study, is that NCI too often gets a blank check from FDA.

Thus, the question Senator Long asks: "Is the FDA hamstringing cancer research?" really ought to be: "Is the FDA hamstringing cancer research by the little, non-government, non-university, non-prestige-hospital men?"

CHAPTER XIV

Dr. Koch's Glyoxylide

Have you ever dreamed of how wonderful it would be if, through some lucky chance, *you* could be the one to discover a cure for cancer? In your dream you are receiving the thanks of the world; governments give you medals, medical societies honor you with citations and testimonials, your respect and honor mount daily in proportion to the gratitude of the world for what you've accomplished. Your final years are spent in golden retirement, surrounded with expressions of the thanks of thousands you've saved from the horrors of cancer.

The alarm that will jolt you out of this reverie is sounded in the new book by Maurice Natenberg entitled, *The Cancer Blackout.* (Published by Regent House, 4554 Broadway, Chicago 40, Ill.) Chances are that after you've read this book you will add a line to your evening prayers, begging that you be left out

[137]

when inspirations for discovering a cancer cure are dispensed. Mr. Natenberg serves up a history which shows that the only governmental recognition likely to come to any one who announces that he has found an effective treatment for cancer is a warning poster on post office billboards; from organized medicine he is likely to see testimonials turned into testimony which will have him disciplined and his discovery discredited; any respect and honor he might have had before he let his findings be known will be swallowed up in bad publicity and vilification; his old age will probably be iron with remorse and bitterness at the thought of having stuck his neck out and ruined his life for nothing, plus the awful frustration of watching deaths mount from a disease he knows he could alleviate. This is the fate that awaits the man who tries to conquer cancer, if past performance is any indication.

That there are men who are willing to face such a prospect is the saving grace of our society. How many more of such men we can hope to see is something else again. Will somebody be successful in introducing an accepted cancer treatment before the hopelessness of it all discourages even the bravest of men? We can only hope so.

Who Are the Discoverers?

In spite of the publicity that would lead one to believe so, the men who have discovered or sponsored treatments for cancer are not all illiterate bumpkins who have a secret poultice to promote, nor are they slickers who would bilk cancer sufferers of their savings to get rich quick. Most are careful scientists whose credits are indicative of the esteem in which they were held before they were seized with this "madness," the desire to do more for cancer victims than surgery and x-ray can do.

Prominent examples of such men are Dr. Walter B. Coffey, who was chief surgeon and director of Southern Pacific Railroad Hospital from 1926 to 1938, and was connected with a cancer treatment known as the Coffey-Humber extract, which was taken from the adrenal cortex of sheep; Dr. William F. Koch, discoverer of Glyoxylide, professor of physiology at Detroit Medical College, 1914-1918, and subject of a laudatory editorial in the *Journal of the American Medical Association* in 1913, heralding his work in endocrinology; Dr. A. C. Ivy, former vice-president of the University of Illinois, original organizer and director of the U.S. Naval Medical Research Institute, recommended by the American Medical Association to represent the Allied governments at the Nuremberg atrocity trials, former executive director of the National Advisory Cancer Society. Can men of such calibre suddenly be labeled crackpots? Can the intelligence which gained them the honor and influence they had be said to have deserted them the minute they began to sponsor a treatment for cancer? Is cancer so hopeless that society brands anyone who would attempt to treat it as demented? It would appear that such is the case.

The stories of Krebiozen, Hoxsey, and Gerson have been told frequently. However, they are only a few in the long trail of frustrating instances in which a promising treatment for cancer was dismissed and its sponsor

[139]

ruined. Mr. Natenberg's book discusses each of the major cancer treatments which have been introduced in the past century. He tells the story of the preparation used and the procedure employed by organized medicine for methodically destroying it. Much to Mr. Natenberg's credit is the method of presentation which is clear and all-inclusive without getting bogged down in such technical talk that the layman is left at the starting gate busily thumbing through a medical dictionary. And the excitement of these stories! You turn page after page convinced that the evidence you've just seen will *have* to draw official approval for this or that treatment. Of course it never happens.

The Story of Glyoxylide

While each one of the stories is interesting, the individual reader is bound to be stirred by one more than another. One of the most arresting is the story of Dr. William Koch's Glyoxylide. This Glyoxylide was a substance designed by Koch to convert the poisons which he believed cause cancer into antitoxins which, by chain reaction, would eliminate the cancerous condition. He used this substance in connection with a rigid diet. Dr. Koch insisted that both must be used, since neither diet nor Glyoxylide would be effective separately.

Dr. Koch was outspoken in his criticism of surgery as a treatment for cancer, and was equally critical of those who promoted surgery in such cases. By public pressure the Wayne County Medical Society of Detroit, Michigan, was forced to initiate an investigation of the Koch treatment. The procedure devised was

[140]

completely fair and thoroughly practical. The only trouble was that the agreed-upon procedure was utterly ignored by the investigators, leaving the result totally inconclusive.

How Dr. Koch's Treatment Was Tested

The plan was this: a group of five physicians would pick cases unknown to Koch to be treated by him. Seven advanced and hopeless cases of internal cancer were selected. So interested was the committee that for three weeks not one member of the committee could be persuaded to certify, officially, that the patients they had chosen had cancer. The patients were getting worse and the longer the delay the more difficult the cure. Dr. Koch then demanded that the head of the medical society direct the committee to perform its duty so that he could begin treatment. The committee examined one, and only one, of the seven patients.

Dr. Koch finally instituted treatment on all seven patients, in order to avoid criticism, without waiting for the committee's examination of the other six. All responded exceedingly well after 3 weeks of treatment. The committee then called the tests off, saying that Koch has refused to cooperate, and they sent the patients home with a warning against continuing Koch's treatment.

The version of the story printed in the *AMA Journal* was in direct contradiction to this and included the accusation that Koch had given only one injection to the patients and simply hadn't bothered to return to continue treatment, so the patients left for home in disgust. Does it seem credible that Koch, after fighting

[141]

for an investigation of his treatment, would abandon his one chance to prove its effectiveness?

Dr. Koch claims the he made every effort to trace the patients but could find only three. All three were able to testify or submit affidavits to the effect that their cancers had been cured.

A Second Hearing

A second hearing was arranged with much difficulty, and in spite of opposition by the AMA Dr. Koch presented a number of patients who had been diagnosed as hopeless and whom he had cured. The committee simply denied both the diagnoses and the cures. In one case a husband testified that his wife had been cured of Paget's disease after she had refused an operation to remove the cancer that had spread from her breast, because it might have meant the loss of her arm. Her surgeon who examined her during the course of her recovery acknowledged in the presence of her husband that she had been cured of cancer. When he was called before the committee, the surgeon testified that his original diagnosis had been falsified and that the woman's condition had really been a simple ulceration, and not cancer at all. He did not say why he had been willing to operate so radically on such a mild condition.

Dr. Koch received several letters of encouragement and expressions of confidence from influential men who sympathized with him because of the unfair treatment he had received at the hands of the committee. Professor W.A. Dewey of the Department of Medicine at the University of Michigan was present at the hearings.

[142]

Of the committee he is quoted as saying, "For a studied intent to falsify, a premeditated determination to condemn everything, and an unscientific, un-American assumption to be judge, jury and prosecuting witness, the report of this so-called committee outstrips in bias, unfairness and mendacity anything that has ever been my lot to observe in a medical practice of forty-four years. . . ."

A vicious campaign against Koch and his formula followed the hearings. Even those who employed Glyoxylide were in danger of losing their professional standing.

Meanwhile, still another cancer investigation was set up, this time in Ontario, Canada. The proceedings were conducted in a dignified and impartial manner. One witness, Dr. J.W. Kannel of Fort Wayne, Indiana, told of treating 72 patients in 14 years with Glyoxylide, due to their own pleadings, though he considered many of these too hopeless to treat in any way. He reported that 21 of these were still alive and four others had died of other causes. Dr. Kannel said that Glyoxylide was the only remedy that had offered him hope in treating cancer, in contrast to his poor results after 24 years of experience with x-ray or radium treatment and surgery. In spite of such impressive evidence no formal report of this hearing was ever published. And that was how the AMA answered queries about its findings. Again an easy way out.

Dr. Koch Disposed Of

In 1942 Dr. Koch was arrested on a charge that his product was falsely labeled. A bail of $10,000 was

[143]

asked, though such a sum is customary only in murder cases. The district attorney admitted that he had asked for the bail on orders from Detroit, to keep Koch from returning to Brazil, where he was then doing research.

Dr. Koch was prosecuted in two more FDA trials concerning Glyoxylide which ended in a permanent injunction against Koch Laboratories. Dr. Koch finally gave up. He assigned the manufacturing process of Glyoxylide to a Detroit religious organization where the preparation was incompletely processed and was no longer effective. Dr. Koch is now living in Brazil and his discovery is no longer in use. Was Glyoxylide really a fraud; or was it an effective treatment for cancer which never got an even break? We will probably never know.

The pattern shown in this case has been repeated time and again in every case of an independent cancer treatment that asked for recognition and approval. The authorities, instead of adhering to principles of investigation which could not be disputed whatever the result, resorted to tricks and vilification of personalities, to inconclusive tests which cast doubt on the outcome, and to hearings whose findings were preordained and whose judges were undeniably biased. As Mr. Natenberg points out, if the medical authorities were as sure of the worthlessness of these treatments as they seemed to be, the fairest and most scrupulous tests by the many experts to whom they have access would only result in the swiftest and most economical proof that the discoverer was promoting a useless product. It is hard to understand why they didn't use that simple tactic, if honest inquiry was their motive.

[144]

CHAPTER XV

Dr. Frost Had A Virus Treatment

In spite of the public picture organized medicine has succeeded in painting of these men, those worth consideration have one thing in common: they invite, they beg for objective evaluation of their work. That is all they ask, and it is the one thing they cannot seem to get. If the medical profession sees fit to pay any attention at all, it is to send a committee whose judgment has been colored by the opinions of colleagues. They will look at the evidence with no great interest and will report that the biopsies were fakes, that cures must be attributed to spontaneous remission or previous treatments, that the patients never really had cancer, or a hundred other accusations and qualifications that would never be applied to a recognized treatment. Of course, with such evaluation the treatment is doomed.

[145]

The developer cries foul, and the medical men point to the committee report, arguing that an evaluation was asked for and given.

Why is an objective evaluation so difficult to achieve? Why can't ground rules be worked out before the inspection begins so that both parties can agree to a plan of procedure and then compare the actual activity to it to see if the rules were obeyed? Then the results would have to be accepted by both parties unless it could be shown that one or the other had deviated from the prescribed plan. Can't Congress formulate reliable ground rules that all would have to obey, so that we could have an accurate picture of the cancer situation and our resources to fight it? We spend millions of dollars yearly on cancer research. Why couldn't some of it be spent, at the insistence of Congress, to investigate claims that an unorthodox cancer cure has been found? The evidence is pretty convincing in some cases. It doesn't seem fair or wise simply to ignore it.

A Non-Conformist

All of this has come out of reading about still another of those hearty, fearless and dedicated men who claims to be able to treat cancer successfully, and has laid his reputation and career on the line to prove it. This time it is Dr. I.N. Frost of Raymondville, Texas. Dr. Frost characterizes himself as a "non-conformist so far as organized medicine is concerned."

It is Dr. Frost's theory that cancer and all other degenerative diseases (ulcer, arthritis, hepatitis, heart disease) are manifestations of a virus infection. His

[146]

treatment begins with a complete reorganization of the diet to include only organically grown food. Then specially developed vaccines are employed, a vaccine made from the patient's own fluids, and one made from the staphylococcus aureus. Along with these, certain antibiotics are used. Dr. Frost, and several others, say the treatment has brought wonderful results.

With this good news to tell, Dr. Frost contacted the local medical societies, inviting them to inspect his formula, his patients and his records. He wrote to 100 local doctors telling them he would like to make a formal report on his results. No reply. He later wrote to the same group volunteering his formula and its schedule of administration. Again no takers. He held 2 public meetings—5 came to one meeting, and none to the other. He wrote a pamphlet describing his work and sent it to the same doctors, but got no response.

That is the way Dr. Frost fought the old accusation that these cancer treatments are secret, but he couldn't even get anyone to listen to him talk about it. Lest he be accused of perfecting a get-rich-quick scheme, Dr. Frost also signed a contract giving all of the money he might collect in the course of treating cancer to a fund for a cancer hospital. He still has no takers.

Aside from his own treatment, he uses the Koch treatment, Krebiozen and Mucorhicin, the Drosnes-Lazenby treatment. He has seen beneficial results from all of these, he says. We presume that the favored treatment varies according to the type of cancer.

It is Dr. Frost's dream to treat 1,000 cancer patients, just after they have gone to the doctor for a checkup

[147]

and learned they have the disease, and who have had no medication, no radiation or surgery, only a proveable diagnosis by biopsy. It is his opinion that he could completely cure at least 800 of the cases, and improve the others in some way.

Do we know if Dr. Frost is truthful and accurate in his claims? We have only his word, and that of some patients who know his work. But, you see, we have no evidence that he is wrong either. Nor has anyone else. We think Dr. Frost and people like him deserve a fair hearing. Why not give him a chance to prove what he says? Why not look at his records, talk to his patients, read their case histories? What is there to be lost?

If the medical profession is sincere in its desire to find a cancer cure, why is it not willing to look for it wherever it might be? Are we to miss it because it occurs in a small laboratory in the southwest instead of the stainless steel and stone skyscraper of a multi-million dollar research center? It is as though we had refused to use electricity because it was discovered by a publisher instead of a scientist, or refused to enjoy the Mona Lisa because it was painted by an inventor, instead of a bona fide artist.

We all know that the good things of this world are rare. It takes talent and courage to produce them. It takes insight, objectivity and courage to find and recognize them. Can we say we are civilized and yet be unwilling to apply these criteria to finding a cure for mankind's most terrible disease?

[148]

CHAPTER XVI

A Doctor's Experience With Krebiozen

An interview with F. Allen Rutherford, M.D.
Lebanon, Pa.

Question: *Doctor, you were one of the leaders of a group who marched on Washington, D.C., in an attempt to convince our Congressmen and government officials of the value of Krebiozen. Why should a man who has had as long and successful a career as you let himself become involved in a cause as unpopular and controversial as Krebiozen?*

Answer: I have seen Krebiozen work. I know that it can achieve beneficial results in the treatment of cancer. Some of my patients are using Krebiozen now, and I am convinced that it is keeping them alive. I could not in good conscience refuse to do everything in my power to see that they have a continuing supply of this lifesaving drug. If this includes involvement in an unpopular and controversial cause, then as a man of conscience I must accept that responsibility.

Q. *How long have you used Krebiozen?*

A. It was about 8½ years ago that I first treated a cancer patient with Krebiozen.

Q. *Was this the first cancer patient you had ever come across in your practice?*

A. Of course not. Up to that time I had any number of patients suffering from cancer. Of these I can recall only two advanced cancer patients who survived more than 5 years under the standard methods of treatment.

Q. *What made you decide to use Krebiozen?*

A. I was dissatisfied with the orthodox methods of treating cancer. I had felt for a long time that there had to be a new approach to the treatment of this disease.

Q. *Would you describe your first experience with Krebiozen? What prompted you to try this new drug?*

A. A former urological patient of mine had cancer of the bladder. He had been under the treatment of several other physicians and surgeons for a period of years. One day his son visited me and told me that his father had just been discharged from a hospital as a terminal case with a life expectance of a mere matter of weeks. He had expressed the desire to see me. As a personal favor to him, I went. I had not seen him for a long time and when I examined him I was certain that he could not survive long. In fact, that same day he had received the last rites of his church. Shortly thereafter, I found in my mail a description of a new anti-cancer drug called Krebiozen being used by Dr.

[150]

Andrew C. Ivy. Now Dr. Ivy's reputation as a scientist in the United States and throughout the world was known to me. His recommendation of the drug awakened my interest. I phoned the son and asked him to my office. I explained in detail the action of Krebiozen so far as I understood it. I asked him if he would be willing to have me try it on his father. The young man agreed. The response was almost miraculous.

Q. *What do you mean by "miraculous?"*

A. Well, he responded immediately, and after five weeks of Krebiozen therapy, he was back at work and worked steadily thereafter. The patient's medical records are available to qualified persons for examination. They show a man whose cancer was deemed incurable and whose physical state was verging on death. This man lived and worked normally for 7 years after his first Krebiozen injection.

Q. *Didn't you hesitate to use the drug for fear of a possible dangerous reaction?*

A. I did not hesitate to use it experimentally when I had the word of Dr. Ivy that the reaction would be non-toxic. My trust has been utterly vindicated. I have never seen, nor do I know of, any toxic effect due to the use of Krebiozen in any patient.

Q. *Do you know of any other cancer drug with a similar record?*

A. I have witnessed the effect of some of the drugs which have been experimentally used in treating cancer and have read reports on others. I know of none that have a non-toxic reaction. Many of them are so toxic that physicians hesitate to use them on even the most

[151]

advanced cancer cases because their effects are as bad as the cancer itself.

Q. *How many patients have you personally treated with Krebiozen?*

A. To date I have treated 298 patients and have set up treatment for about 50 or so others. In the latter cases, the patients' own personal physicians continued the Krebiozen treatment which had been initiated by me.

Q. *Would you describe the condition of the patients who come to you?*

A. About 97 per cent of the cancer patients who come to me for Krebiozen therapy are and have been far advanced or terminal cases, considered hopeless by their attending physicians. In fact, in some cases I have been called in at the last moment when their condition was so critical that nothing could be done, due to the widespread metastases, other than to relieve their pain.

One in Eight Helped

Q. *How many of the patients you have treated with Krebiozen have been helped?*

A. About one in eight have shown a favorable response.

Q. *What do you call a "favorable response?"*

A. A reduction of pain which occurs in about 50 per cent of the cases, and a prolongation of life, with the cancer arrested or controlled.

Q. *What type of cancer can be treated with Krebiozen?*

A. I have treated about 35 different types of malig-

[152]

nancy involving practically every part of the body and occurring in every age group from 3½ to 83 years.

Q. *Do cancer patients who consult you ask specifically for treatment with Krebiozen?*

A. I receive hundreds of letters from cancer patients and their relatives and friends all over the country, asking me to treat them with Krebiozen, or to recommend a doctor who will do so in their own locality. All patients who come to my office for treatment of cancer ask me to use Krebiozen.

Q. *Can you estimate for yourself the probable effect of Krebiozen on a patient after having examined him?*

A. I cannot. There is no way to predict the effects of Krebiozen on any type of cancer, as it would be impossible to presume that it will work in one case and not another.

Q. *As a physician, have you ever been surprised at Krebiozen's effect on a patient?*

A. This happens many times. Some patients come to me and after examining them I am reluctant to begin treatment because I am doubtful that anything can help them due to widespread metastases. Yet oftentimes Krebiozen will have a beneficial effect by arresting growth. Then there are patients who I feel will be benefitted greatly, and after several months of treatment I am unfortunately proven wrong.

Q. *Do you believe that other forms of treatment offer a firmer ground for predicting the results of the treatment than Krebiozen does?*

A. Positively not. No doctor can predict the effect

[153]

of his treatment of a cancer with any certainty. If we could, cancer would be much less of a problem than it is now. Surgeons can only hope that their operations will be effective in removing the cancer; radiologists can only hope that they have been able to burn out the cancerous areas; doctors who inject various chemicals can only hope that the cancer will be eradicated before the patient dies. None of them can look at a patient and say with any surety that the treatment they plan to use will be effective.

No Cure Promised

Q. *What do you tell your patients about the chances of a cure?*

A. I never use the term "cure" in relation to a cancer treatment. I tell the patients that I believe Krebiozen offers them hope. I tell them this because I do have that conviction. I tell them that they have a good chance of ridding themselves of their pain, and that the treatment holds the best possibility I know of to prolong their lives and their usefulness to their families and themselves.

Q. *How long does the treatment with Krebiozen take?*

A. I have no way of predicing how much treatment will be required for an individual case. It varies as in other forms of therapy. There are many factors which are involved, such as grade, location, and extent of metastases. Some require more frequent injections and larger doses of Krebiozen, and might require a long continuance of the therapy. Some patients have taken it for five or more years.

Q. *Can you give an estimation of the average number of injections of Krebiozen needed as maintenance dosage?*

A. Many of my patients are on maintenance doses of Krebiozen twice monthly. Some require Krebiozen once a week and some require injections even more frequently. I cannot say what an "average" would be. It depends entirely on the individual case.

Q. *How much does Krebiozen cost the patient?*

A. Krebiozen is supplied by Promak Laboratories, producers of Krebiozen and the production cost is $9.50 per ampule. However, the doctor is informed that if his patient is unable to contribute the full cost of production and the case is considered worthwhile for clinical investigation, the amount which the patient can afford to contribute will be left to the judgment of his physician and the patient. The Krebiozen Research Foundation is then informed of the individual situation and the case is considered for partial or complete charity distribution. I have frequently had patients who were unable to pay for their treatment at all and the drug was supplied to them at absolutely no cost.

There was a time when there was no charge for Krebiozen at all but the producers have found it impossible to continue experimental work on the drug without meeting the very expensive costs of production, through some outside source. Without these contributions, these supplies of Krebiozen would be almost impossible to produce, financially speaking.

[155]

Conspiracy?

Q. *Do you believe that there is a conspiracy to keep Krebiozen off the market, even though the conspirators are convinced of its ability to act favorably on cancer?*

A. I do.

Q. *Why would anyone thwart a treatment for cancer? Doctors have friends and relatives suffering from the disease too. It seems that they as much as anyone else would want to see to the availability of a successful treatment.*

A. Quite right, but the thousands of doctors in practice have very little say in making a policy. These doctors are dependent upon the AMA to make a policy for them to follow, and they follow it. The average doctor believes what the AMA tells him to believe. About Krebiozen, the AMA has told him to believe it is a fraud.

Q. *If the AMA's attitude towards Krebiozen is not based on an honest evaluation of the drug, what is your explanation for the AMA's policy against this drug?*

A. When Krebiozen was first introduced, an officer of the AMA tried to get the sales rights with a view to the profits that lay in effective anti-cancer drugs. Krebiozen's developer, Stevan Durovic, M.D., refused a financial deal and because of it was threatened with ruin. Dr. Andrew C. Ivy who did much of the subsequent research and testing of Krebiozen, was threatened with professional embarrassment and harassment unless he would revoke his endorsement of Krebiozen. The refusal of both of these men to cooperate with the

[156]

then officer of the AMA, lies at the root of Krebiozen's troubles.

The deliberate inaccuracy in the AMA's first reports on Krebiozen began a campaign of vilification against the drug and its sponsors which has continued until this very day. The AMA cannot easily reverse its stand on Krebiozen, in view of all of the groundwork that has been done to discredit the drug, without losing face with its membership, and with the American public.

Government Agencies

Q. *What about the government agencies such as the FDA and the National Cancer Institute? Why have they made it so difficult for Krebiozen to obtain a double-blind test that will either expose the drug as a fraud, or give it to the world as a safe, effective cancer treatment?*

A. Who do you suppose controls the decision on a question such as this?—Experts recruited from the high echelons of the AMA, of course. Politicians, who have no medical background, look for an opinion as to whether Krebiozen is worth the testing. To whom do you suppose they look for such an opinion?—Doctors who represent the AMA, of course. What verdict would one expect from these doctors but "no?"

I assure you that if the outcome of the double-blind test on Krebiozen were expected by them to prove that the drug is a fraud, the test would be set up tomorrow. The doctors are well aware, however, that Krebiozen is safer and more effective than any of the other anti-cancer drugs which have been tested and pushed by

[157]

representatives of the AMA and executives of large pharmaceutical companies. How will these people look to the American public when it is shown that the one drug they suppressed for almost a decade is the only one which stands out favorably? A review of the facts indicates that the various organized groups purporting to seek a cure for cancer, including Federal government agencies such as the HEW, NCI and the FDA, do not really welcome any cancer remedy which they themselves have not subsidized. In the case of Krebiozen, there is more than professional jealousy involved.

Q. *How do you account for the many anti-cancer drugs which do get a test by government agencies?*

A. The very circumstances which have created Krebiozen's problems are the ones which open the doors for other drugs.

The government earmarks millions yearly for research to produce a drug which will successfully treat cancer. The drug companies vie for a slice of these millions. When they come up with something they think might work, they submit it to the National Cancer Institute for testing at government expense. It is a foregone conclusion that a drug developed at government expense will be accepted for testing by the National Cancer Institute. Furthermore, it should be realized that any patent for a drug successfully used to treat cancer is worth millions. The drug company which gets an OK on a cancer drug is bound to be "very grateful" to anyone who had anything to do with its acceptance.

[158]

Remember again that AMA representatives are on the boards which advise the government where to put its research money. AMA representatives are on the boards of the government agencies which test the drugs as they are developed. AMA representatives are also on the boards of directors of the large drug companies. It would indicate that the AMA is part of a conspiracy against Krebiozen, and it is also part of the strong conspiracy in favor of other drugs developed by large corporations. One need only review the recent scandals in the Food and Drug Administration, the Welch case in particular, to realize that this fantastic situation is all too real!

Q. *We hear the charge that only the poor and deluded are naive enough to seek Krebiozen as a cancer treatment. Would you give us an idea of the economic and intellectual range of your patients?*

A. I have treated a U.S. senator, a brother of one, and a son of a former one. Nurses, ministers, educators, businessmen, the wealthy and the poor, have sought Krebiozen therapy either for themselves of for members of their families.

Nurses have recommended Krebiozen therapy. They are good judges of the value of a given therapy. Their recommendation alone should give the drug special consideration.

Q. *Critics of Krebiozen frequently state that persons seemingly cured through the use of the drug never really had cancer. Is it possible that cancers which have responded to Krebiozen were never really cancer at all?*

[159]

A. Of course all things are possible but this circumstance is highly improbable. This criticism is also applicable to the so-called cures of orthodox therapy. When a patient consults me, a biopsy and/or X-ray findings are requested. If the experts who make the diagnoses err, then the mistake is not mine. These patients had been treated for cancer by other physicians who had also accepted the experts' diagnoses.

I assure you that if a Krebiozen treated cancer patient were to die rather than recover, the cause of death would have been unhesitatingly certified as cancer.

So you see the charge is one that is easily disproved. The records of the patients who have been treated and responded to Krebiozen are available for examination by any qualified person.

Q. *What of the recent charge that Drs. Ivy and Durovic refused to cooperate in furnishing required data to the various government agencies?*

A. My congressman, Representative Kunkle, informed me in Washington that this charge was retracted. However, while the accusation received nationwide coverage, no retraction has been noted in newspapers by any of my patients or myself.

Q. *Is Krebiozen a secret treatment? This is a charge that is frequently used as a reason for not testing Krebiozen.*

A. There is no secret about the content of Krebiozen. A full chemical analysis has been submitted to the authorities several times. It is considered to be a local hormone or "autocoid." Its empirical formula is $C_{25}H_{67}N_{18}O_{19}$ with a molecular weight of 923.93. About

[160]

10 mgs. of crystalline Krebiozen was sent to the NCI as a proof that it exists and is not just mineral oil as its detractors claim.

Of course, until the developers of the drug are fully protected with a patent, the method for producing the drug cannot be divulged. If it were divulged before a patent is granted, there would be no way to protect the investment of time and money made by Krebiozen's developers against hundreds of large and small drug companies who might try to duplicate their feat. In fact, it is known that three such attempts are now in progress.

Q. *Just what effects do you see in patients who respond to Krebiozen?*

A. I see patients who were in agony sit up and begin to enjoy the world around them. I see people who have been given up as hopeless, miraculously recover. I see them return to jobs, become housekeepers again, gain weight, rekindle their interest in social activities, and regain a normal outlook. Of course, this does not happen in every case, but it does happen often enough to make me glad that I am enabled to use it. Krebiozen takes up where surgery and radiation let go. And best of all, it is non-toxic.

Q. *How do the patients feel about Krebiozen while they are in the process of treatment?*

A. I think the best answer to that question is the fact that more than a hundred patients being treated with Krebiozen recently gathered in Washington from all parts of the country to protest the threatened loss of this drug through red tape and manipulation of the

[161]

law. Threatened with the possibility that availability of Krebiozen might be halted, these patients are convinced that any chance they have for recovery or even control of their disease would be halted too. Krebiozen to them is what insulin is to the diabetic.

Q. *Since you have become involved in the Krebiozen controversy, have you experienced any repercussions in your own career?*

A. Since my involvement with Krebiozen, there have been few days *without* repercussions to my career. I have been called a quack and a racketeer. I have been charged falsely with demanding and receiving exorbitant fees. I was banned from practicing in my local hospital. At first, when I was reinstated at the hospital, nurses were ordered to refuse me clinical assistance. I have been ostracized by my colleagues. I have been professionally harassed in one way or another since I began to state loud and clear that I believe in Krebiozen and use it.

Fortunately for me, this situation has occurred during the last days of my long medical career. I feel that my reputation has been established too long to be seriously damaged. After all, I am a past president of my county medical society. I have taught medicine at one of the finest medical schools in the country. I also aided in a research project for a large pharmaceutical firm.

I refused to budge from my conviction that Krebiozen is valuable in the treatment of cancer. A younger man who has a career yet to carve in the medical world might be intimidated by the things

[162]

which have happened to me and I could hardly blame him. I, however, will not be intimidated.

Other Measures Taken

Q. *When you give Krebiozen, is that the total extent of your treatment and your advice to the patient?*

A. No. I believe that Krebiozen can act alone as a therapy. However, I do believe that there is better chance for the patient's recovery if he will help himself. By helping himself, I mean that he should refrain entirely from smoking and drinking. I believe that he should embark on a diet which does not contain carcinogens (cancer-producing agents). Special attention should be directed towards correcting all abnormal body functions.

Q. *Would you describe in general the type of diet you recommend?*

A. The type of diet depends upon the location of the cancer. The amounts of fats and proteins may be limited. Fresh fruits and vegetables and their juices are considered important.

Many ordinary food items are not included in the diet because they are considered to be harmful.

Each patient receives a diet according to his special needs.

Q. *Do you use any other drugs aside from Krebiozen?*

A. Yes, for complications. For example, antibiotics for infections, diuretics for edema, etc. And where narcotics are necessary, I try to replace them with non-narcotics. But I use these drugs only so long as they

[163]

are absolutely necessary. I watch the patient closely for the first signs that will allow me to discontinue their use. This is my attitude in general toward all drugs.

Q. *Doctor, would you care to state your opinion as to just what cancer really is?*

A. I believe that cancer is due to a faulty cellular chemistry that has been produced by trauma, either physical or chemical. In cancer, cellular activity is stimulated to a point at which there is no longer a normal control. The cell activity goes haywire. In cancer, the cells multiply and increase in size to a point at which they form a tumor or replace cells which have a definite function in preserving the integrity of the body's health.

It is true that normal body repair stimulates cell activity but this activity is self-limiting. In normal wound repair the body works to produce an increased number of cells so that scar tissue is formed to cover the wound. But you will notice that the excess activity stops when the point has been reached at which repair is complete. The normal body does not continue cell manufacture so that the scar tissue would form a lump at the site of the wound. Proper cellular chemistry controls this amazing faculty. It seems to me that faulty cellular chemistry might be responsible for abusing it.

Q. *What do you think of the current theory that a virus is the cause of cancer?*

A. I am not convinced that a virus is the cause of cancer because cancer does not have the symptoms of an infection produced by micro-organisms.

[164]

Q. *What are Krebiozen's chances of acceptance by orthodox practitioners?*

A. I am convinced that if more physicians could see the results of Krebiozen treatment generally, they would accept it. Some doctors have been so intimidated by what has happened to other practitioners who use Krebiozen that they are afraid to try it. Others, acting upon the advice and opinion of the American Medical Association, refuse to have any contact whatsoever with Krebiozen. There are, however, a number of doctors throughout the United States who use Krebiozen and have found it effective in treating their patients. Some of them even use it secretively, rather than face the repercussions that are likely to come their way. I can tell you that there are some doctors who have themselves been treated with Krebiozen. If I or any member of my family contracted cancer, I would certainly use it. In fact, at present, I am treating my niece with Krebiozen.

Q. *Would you care to speculate on when, if ever, the much-publicized double-blind test of Krebiozen by the National Cancer Institute will be made?*

A. I believe that the possibilties of this test being done lie to a great extent in the hands of the public. If there were enough public indignation registered with the legislators whose responsibility it is to see that such public institutions are run for the benefit of the taxpayers, we might have a chance.

As I stated before, the *"lipo-sac"* theory is being explored by other scientists. It is therefore quite possible that an effort will be made to delay such a

[165]

test of Krebiozen until after a duplicate has been made, tested, and approved. Then Krebiozen can be labeled as a poor substitute for the approved horse serum drug. I hope this does not occur for this would be a travesty of justice for the scientists who have labored so long and endured the vilification of their detractors.

The quicker the test for Krebiozen can be agreed upon and completed, the better the chance that Krebiozen will be recognized as the valuable therapy it is. Only public demand can speed this development. Letters to congressmen, and to influential figures throughout the country from your readers and anyone else of influence will be most helpful to this cause.

I am grateful to you for this opportunity to present my views on Krebiozen therapy and the issues involved.

Note: *Shipment of Krebiozen in interstate commerce has been banned by the Food and Drug Administration. At present, it is only in the state of Illinois that any Krebiozen therapy for cancer is being carried on.*

[166]

CHAPTER XVII

The Gerson Treatment:
Quackery or
Suppressed Science?

In 1954 doctors advised Joe Panebianco, stricken with lung cancer, to take his long-desired trip to Florida because it appeared that he might have only days to live. In 1958, Joe was happily managing his bicycle shop in New Jersey.

Extensive skin cancer forced doctors to remove the nose of a New York clergyman in 1949. Five months later, the mucous membranes improved so much that a plastic nose could be built. In 1954, the patient had reported no further relapses and was still working.

These are only two of many people, who, doomed to pain and death, have found renewed comfort and life. They were lucky enough to have heard of Max Gerson, M.D., a German-born doctor who discovered a dietary treatment for a type of skin tuberculosis in 1929. Arriving in America in 1936, he brought with him another dietary "cure"—this time for cancer. His clinic in Nanuet, New York, claimed considerable success in curing, without surgery or radiation, cancers of the skin, esophagus, liver, bone, lung, breast, stomach and brain in terminal cases given up by doctors.

The clinic was in operation until 1958, the year before Dr. Gerson died of pneumonia.

Essentially, the accepted treatment of cancer has not changed in the last 20 years. Of three types of treatment recognized by the medical fraternity: surgery, radiation and certain approved drugs, a doctor must select one when cancer is diagnosed. Then he might have to try another, and finally the third. More than this he must not do, unless he is willing to risk trouble with the local medical fraternity. It is the doctor's grim task, after the last operation or drug has been tried, to tell the patient there is no hope. The patient is expected to accept this verdict and try to pay his doctor and hospital bills before he dies.

Some patients are not willing to bow out so gracefully. The prospect of dying arouses a determination in them to seek help in a new direction. Some of them try the Gerson treatment for cancer. Some of those who do, recover.

Dr. Gerson's Record

The Gerson treatment for cancer is not a new one. Even before coming to the United States from Germany in 1936, Dr. Max Gerson developed a therapy, basically dietetic, to treat various diseases, including cancer. Eventually he concentrated on treating cancer in a small sanitarium (closed at Dr. Gerson's death from pneumonia in 1959), in Nanuet, New York. The proportion of his successes with patients who had been designated as terminal cases by their family doctors and specialists, was impressive. For many of them merely to remain alive for several months was a triumph. When these same patients found themselves freed from pain and able to enjoy happy, productive lives, the only accurate description for them was "phenomenal."

A visit to Nanuet in 1957 by a member of *Prevention's* staff convinced her that Dr. Gerson was indeed having success in treating cancer. She spoke to patients who were themselves sure they had been cured, and had x-rays to prove it. One of them, a woman, had seen her cancer of the spine disappear. Five years after her treatment under Gerson, the woman who had come to Nanuet from Chicago for a check-up was well —"strong enough to move a piano," said Gerson.

There was a man there who came to Dr. Gerson afflicted with a cancerous stomach and a cancerous bladder. He had been told by his doctors that he couldn't hope to live much more than six weeks. Three weeks under the Gerson treatment had led to remarkable improvement in his condition. After seven months the cancer was gone.

These stories were not new ones to Dr. Gerson. He had been successful many times in restoring hopeless cancer patients to health. He wrote a book (*A Cancer Therapy—Results of 50 Cases*) which described in detail 50 case histories of patients whose cancers had responded to his treatment. Among them were malignant brain tumors, cancer of the upper spinal cord, abdominal cancer, lung cancer, cancer of the breast, of the ovaries, of the testicle, of the lymph glands and of the bone. Just about every major cancer type was included with full documentation and history from previous treatment.

Because of the book the Gerson treatment is available to any physician who might be otherwise forced to tell a cancer patient there is no hope after surgery, radiation or drugs. Yet, most doctors advise their patients to wait for death rather than use the Gerson method for treating cases. We find it hard to understand why.

Restoring Normal Metabolism

The method is simple enough. Basically it is aimed at restoring the body's chemistry to normalcy through diet. In Dr. Gerson's words, "There is no cancer in a normal metabolism . . . the liver is the center of the restoration process in those patients who improve strikingly. If the liver is too destroyed, then the treatment cannot be effective. . . . It is generally known that in cancer, especially in advanced cases, all the various metabolic systems are impaired."

Dr. Gerson believed that the metabolism of sodium and potassium, especially, is important in treating cancer patients. "Diet and medication serve the purpose of restoring potassium and the minerals of the potassium group to the tissues until they are completely saturated, and, conversely reconveying sodium and its group out of the cells into the circulatory fluids, the connective tissues and other tissues where they belong. The retentive surplus of sodium must be eliminated. It is only on that basis that further recovery of the organs can take place," wrote Dr. Gerson.

To accomplish this the patient is put on a very strict diet, low in animal protein, high in vegetables and fruits. There must be no alcohol, coffee, tobacco, no refined, canned or frozen foods, no foods processed in any way at all. The patient may not have any white flour or white sugar, or anything made from them. No fats, no oils, no salt substitutes are permitted.

Fresh Foods

The food the patient does eat may not be prepared in a pressure cooker or an aluminum utensil. Fresh-squeezed fruit and vegetable juices, as well as raw liver juice make up an important part of the Gerson patient's diet. Along with these, much fruit, especially apples, (the berry fruits are not considered desirable), and many vegetables, particularly carrots, celery, greens and potatoes, help to fill in the diet. Oatmeal and whole rye bread are also allowed.

As the patient shows improvement, certain types of food are restored to the diet. Protein allowances begin after the first few weeks with cheese and fish in small amounts. Eventually a full but careful natural diet is achieved. Organically grown foods are recommended for fullest success. (When an effort is being made to eliminate poisons from the body, it hardly makes sense to introduce new ones in the form of residues of insecti-

[171]

cides and additives in the food one eats. However, the Gerson treatment has had its successes even when organic food was not available.)

To speed the initial cleansing of the body from its poisons, the Gerson treatment calls for frequent enemas —several a day in the beginning—until the body begins to show some effective opposition to the cancer. Along with this, thyroid, lugol solution and 10 per cent potassium solution, acidol pepsin capsules, lubile capsules and a 10 per cent solution of caffeine potassium citrate plus injections of vitamin B and liver, fill out the basic Gerson treatment.

Dr. Gerson believed that the chemical and artificial treatment of the soil deprives us of greatly needed natural elements. For this reason, the dietary treatment consists of organic foods to fortify the liver, which in turn is believed better able to combat the unnatural condition of cancerous cells. In his book, *A Cancer Therapy: Results of Fifty Cases* Dr. Gerson wrote: "For the benefit of coming generations, I think it is high time we change our agriculture and food preservation methods. . . . The coming years will make it more and more imperative that organically grown fruits and vegetables will be, and must be, used for protection against degenerative diseases, the prevention of cancer, and more so in treatment of cancer."

The writings of Dr. Gerson always emphasized that this drastic treatment was designed specifically for cancerous conditions, and was by no means to be used as preventive therapy by a healthy person. He also warned that his method could not guarantee complete

[172]

recovery for every case. Dr. Gerson believed that a patient cannot treat himself at home alone, since medication and diet must be adapted to individual needs. In addition, another person must be available to administer enemas and to provide a constant supply of nourishment from a busy kitchen. Yet, even the expectation of some physical discomfort and exertion did not discourage a large number of patients from besieging the already filled-to-capacity clinic.

Some Drop Out

The diet is difficult to follow. The timing for drinking the juices (always freshly squeezed) and for taking the enemas and shots, literally consumes most of one's waking hours. Unless the patient is completely ambulatory, he must have full-time assistance. It is this circumstance, more than any other, which causes some patients to stop the treatment. They say they simply can't do it.

It is hard to predict what one would or would not do under particular circumstances. Who can say that he would surely stay with the diet? But remember, this is a diet for curing cancer! If it were a case of keeping the diet or dying, could anything be too much trouble?

Cancer patients are haunted by a problem that is almost as hard to cope with as the disease itself: where is the money to come from? Estimates are given which set $6,000 as the average amount of money a cancer patient spends on medical care before he dies. By the time most patients decide on the Gerson treatment, they are close to, if not in excess of, the $6,000 average.

[173]

What more can they expect in expenses if they agree to the Gerson treatment?

What It Costs

The Gerson treatment costs can be approximated by knowing that the initial visit includes a complete physical examination, some tests, the taking of a detailed history, and a full explanation of the schedule and diet which must be followed. This requires about 2 or 3 hours. Laboratory tests of the blood, etc., are carried out by a commercial laboratory. Certain of these may have to be repeated in the course of the treatment.

The patient must have a reamer type juicer, which, if electric, can cost as much as $300. Future visits to the doctor are usually scheduled for 4 weeks after the initial visit then every one to three months for the duration of the treatment, except in case of emergency. The physician's fee and the cost of laboratory tests, we assume, must vary with the individual physician, laboratory and locality. The recommended time of treatment is 18 months.

The medications are not expensive. The foods can be —especially if one cannot grow one's own organic foods. The estimate we received from such a patient was $35 per week spent on foods for her diet. Of course, season and location influence this cost appreciably.

Gerson a Quack?

There is no secret in the Gerson treatment. It seems to be at least as effective as the best anti-cancer measures subscribed to by the American Medical Association. It is safer than any of them and cheaper than most of them. The recovery rate was claimed to be as high or higher. Yet we can find few doctors who approve of it, and fewer yet who will use it. They say Dr. Gerson was a quack, a charlatan.

Dr. Gerson was a recognized medical expert in Europe and had published many papers on cancer in Germany's leading professional journals. A few years after coming to the United States he was invited by the U. S. Senate to give expert testimony in hearings of 1946 which were aimed at a coordinated effort by "the world's outstanding experts . . . to discover means of curing and preventing cancer." It was the first time in history that the senate had honored a physician in this way. Certainly he was a man of stature in medicine.

Before Dr. Gerson came to this country, his reputation was highly esteemed by such honored men as the late Dr. Albert Schweitzer. American medicine preferred to ignore the evidence of cured cases presented in Senate hearings and illustrative literature. Although the clinic claimed to have cured patients of cancer, the extent of such claims remains unconfirmed because no one was willing to investigate. Today, the Foundation for Cancer Treatment, Inc., established by a number of grateful patients to continue the publication of his teachings, has dropped out of existence for sheer lack of interest.

It is disheartening to learn that few doctors today will even attempt to treat cancer patients with the relatively safe Gerson method. Instead, the higher-cost-

[175]

ing conventional surgery, radiation or approved drugs are used exclusively even when it may be known that such treatments have come too late. The situation might change, however, if doctors were persuaded to read *A Cancer Therapy*, which describes the favorable results from treating 50 different types of cancer by the Gerson method. The details of the technique are so thoroughly explained that a qualified doctor could administer the treatment.

Others on Same Track

Although the abundant literature about and by Dr. Gerson has made him quite well known, he was not the only one to consider cancer the result of improper nutrition and metabolism. The late Dr. John Davidson of Winnipeg, Manitoba, also believed that cancer is a nutritional deficiency disease. His treatment, reported able to halt the spread of human cancer, was similar to Dr. Gerson's, but rare beef, a preparation from chick embryos, and massive doses of vitamins from cod liver oil, brewer's yeast, and wheat germ oil were included.

Another interesting observation was reported in the *Journal of Proctology* (Feb., 1961). Dr. Donald C. Collins mentioned 5 people who were diagnosed as cancer cases, but were cured by eating organically grown foods. He stated: "The only constant factor in the lives of these 5 persons was the fact that they all ate home-raised, organically grown foods that were free from chemical preservatives and insect repellent sprays."

Treatments employed by quacks and charlatans are

often kept secret because to reveal them would be to reveal their worthlessness. The Gerson treatment for cancer has been published by Dr. Gerson himself in minute detail. It has appeared in many other publications. Its theory is scientifically plausible, with particular references to the operation of the body's chemistry. Many scientists agree with Dr. Gerson that the ability of the liver to function properly, and a breakdown of over-all metabolism is basically involved with the cancer problem. Restoring these functions is a difficult accomplishment. Dr. Gerson seems to have found a safe, effective way to do it. We see no reason why orthodoxy should be a requirement in a successful cancer treatment. Orthodoxy seems to lead to more blind alleys than it does to successes.

Quacks and charlatans prey on helpless victims and bleed them of their last cent. Dr. Gerson could hardly have hoped to become wealthy through using his method. The periodic examinations are widely spaced. The drugs are simple and inexpensive. The chemical tests can be done by any reliable commercial laboratory at a competitive price. The foods, of course, are bought from any source for organically raised foods available. A quack would surely invent a more lucrative type of treatment than this.

Why the Opposition?

Why then has the Gerson method for cancer treatment had such tough sledding? Why does organized medicine oppose its use? A newspaper reporter, S. J. Haught, in the book, *Cancer Cure?* (London Press, No.

[177]

Hollywood, California), describes the frustration he experienced in trying to get the answer to this question. At every turn he was met with a solid wall of contradiction. A letter to the American Medical Association brought the reply that . . . "although Dr. Gerson had been requested to do so, he had failed or refused to acquaint the medical profession with the details of his treatment." Dr. Gerson attempted to publish his findings in several American medical journals to no avail. There are rejection letters to prove it. Yet he had published 50 medical papers in Europe with no trouble at all. The refusal "to acquaint the medical profession with the details of his treatment" could hardly be said to be his.

Dr. Gerson was suspended "from the rights and privileges of membership" by the Medical Society of the County of New York "as a result of personal publicity." The occasion of this infraction of the society's ill-defined ethical rules was an appearance on an all-night spontaneous discussion program on a New York radio station. They discussed the Gerson treatment, naturally. For his part in the discussion, Dr. Gerson was suspended. The program had had other M.D.'s who discussed a wide variety of medical subjects and techniques in which they were knowledgeable or proficient. Their salvation lay in first acquiring permission from the MSCNY to appear. This Dr. Gerson failed to do. Still, this infraction was a rather tenuous reason for discrediting a world renowned physician who might have the answer to cancer.

It seems ludicrous to report that Dr. Gerson had

[178]

trouble because, it was alleged, he was unwilling to make public his method. Then, to report in the next paragraph that an all-night broadcast during which his method was openly described and discussed for hours, brought down the medical society's wrath because of too much publicity. But those are the facts.

Mr. Haught tells us that no official evaluation of the Gerson treatment has ever been revealed by his medical colleagues, although Dr. Gerson submitted to 5 investigations of his patients and their records by the Medical Society of the County of New York. Neither Dr. Gerson, nor anyone else, has ever been able to learn the results of any of those investigations. If the results are as damning as we are led to believe, why not tell the world?

The Gerson case is another of those mysteries which surround the tight core of American medical orthodoxy. Doctors treating cancer perform operations they know will be useless. They use drugs whose side effects are recognized as deadly, with full A. M. A. approval. They prescribe radiation which is likely to cause one cancer in the process of treating another. All this will bring no objection from a medical society. But if a doctor uses a diet rich in nutrients on the theory that a healthy body can fight its own way out of cancer, he can expect big trouble.

We do not say that the Gerson treatment will improve or cure every cancer patient. Even doctors using the method don't make any such claims. But something happens to many of the patients under his treatment which has them walking, working and living for

[179]

years after they were judged by specialists to be beyond help of the orthodox treatment. How can it be reasonable to condemn the use of Gerson's method even for a terminal cancer patient?

How Many Could be Helped?

It is impossible to estimate how many successes the Gerson treatment would have if it were used on the grand scale of the accepted cancer treatments. But consider that Dr. Gerson was able to include 50 case histories of successful treatment of *different types* of cancer in his book. Many of these were rare and hopeless cases. Most of them had tried everything else to no avail. If one man could produce such a record from his own experience, imagine what results could be achieved if the system were used throughout the country by a large number of physicians, on patients whose cancer had not been permitted to progress to the point of despair.

The ghost of Dr. Max Gerson hangs over the entire question of cancer research today. Why he was not accepted by American medicine we cannot say. He may have made mistakes in trying to introduce his revolutionary treatment to a new country. Perhaps he unwittingly antagonized influential men. The radio program might have been extremely ill-advised from a professional point of view. If any one of these brought down the wrath of organized medicine, none of them should matter now. The only question to be resolved is this: can the Gerson treatment reverse the course of cancer? Many believe the answer is frequently yes.

CHAPTER XVIII

A Treatment Ignored to Death

Two English researchers have a theory that the ever-increasing use of antibiotics may have a lot to do with the rising incidence of cancer; Dr. B. A. Meyer and Dr. J. D. Benjafield of the staff of St. George's Hospital, London, have written in *The Medical Press* for August 31, 1955, "Antibiotics are by far the greatest life-saving discovery in the history of medicine, and most of the antibiotics are relatively innocuous when compared with antiseptics, but it seems that a minority of patients are sensitive or allergic to some of them. The impairment of their therapeutic value through reckless and indiscriminate use is a very serious matter, for they are too frequently given for mild infections such as coughs, colds, coryza, sinusitis, and many other respiratory infections, no matter how trivial they may be. Patients often demand penicillin injections from their doctors, and many a doctor is forced to give them lest he should offend the patient and be thought not to be keeping abreast of modern methods."

They go on to say that none of the present-day anti-

[181]

biotics apparently has any effect against viruses. If, as some researchers believe, cancer is due to a virus, may it not be possible that, by damaging the tissues in some subtle manner, the antibiotics may upset the body's natural ability to create immunity to viruses? This ability has been acquired and perfected through millions of years and it seldom fails. But if cancer is caused by a virus and if the antibiotics have destroyed the body's power against viruses, then might we not conclude that antibiotics have a lot to do with increased cancer rates?

Since antibiotics were introduced, deaths from lung cancer shot up by more than 140 per cent in this country, although the mortality from other forms of cancer increased only 31 per cent. "Recent statistics again show that town dwellers are more affected by carcinoma of the lung than rural dwellers. On the other hand, the primitive races in Africa and Asia show no increase in the incidence of cancer. Is it not true that town dwellers have better facilities for medical treatment and that since antibiotics are in vogue they are freely given?" ask the two researchers. "In rural areas, owing to shortage of medical personnel, antibiotics are given much less freely. Among the primitive races of Africa and Asia medical facilities are so few that there is very limited application of antibiotics."

Since antibiotics disturb the delicate relationship between bacteria and viruses they must definitely interfere with the defensive mechanism of the body, say Drs. Meyer and Benjafield. Of course there are other differences between rural and city dwellers, as other

[182]

researchers have pointed out. There is more air pollution in cities. Country folks generally get a lot more healthful outdoor exercise in clean air. So far as primitive peoples in Africa and Asia are concerned, they are not exposed to the flood of refined, lifeless, over-chemicalized food that is practically the only food available for "civilized" people. However, we must not discount the truth of Meyer's and Benjafield's statements about antibiotics.

Dr. Meyer's Book Explains the Theory in Full

Dr. Meyer, with another colleague, Dr. Irene Orgel, has written a book called *The Cancer Patient* (published by J. and A. Churchill, 1950) in which they outline a cancer treatment for advanced cases. They do not advocate their "chemotherapy" as they call it, as a cancer cure, though in some hopeless cases they have been able to prolong the patient's life by five years and more of happy useful existence—but rather they advocate their method for enabling those afflicted with cancer to end their lives free from pain, free from fear and free from the kind of state induced by morphine and other powerful painkillers.

They tell us in this book that for some reason or other cancer patients cannot use vitamin C as healthy persons do. The cancer cell, suffering from an injury to a certain apparatus within the cell, cannot adequately use the vitamin C it absorbs and so it absorbs more and more from the tissues in an effort to maintain itself. The patient becomes deficient in vitamin C and the vitamin accumulates at the site of the cancer.

[183]

There is a lowered vitamin C level in other diseases, too—rheumatoid arthritis and congestive heart failure, for instance. But in no other disease is the finding so constant as in cancer, Drs. Meyer and Orgel tell us. The same is true of guinea pigs with cancer. Their store of the vitamin is exhausted far more readily than is that of normal animals.

Interestingly enough, the adrenal glands of cancer patients have been found to contain far less vitamin C than those of normal people. The adrenal glands are those mechanisms of the body which protect us against shock and injury. *The hormone or substance manufactured by one part of the adrenal glands is also concerned with controlling growth.* Could it be that lack of vitamin C in the cancer patient, by disrupting this growth hormone, may contribute to the spread of the cancer?

Dr. Meyer and Dr. Orgel experimented with a preparation in which they combined vitamin C with minerals in such a way as to make the cancer tissues take up and use the vitamin C. This, they believed, would adjust the metabolism of the malignant cells so that they would stop extracting more and more vitamin C from the blood. Then the level of vitamin C in other parts of the body would be raised. The vitamin store in the adrenal glands would be replaced and the patient would feel better.

They combined zinc and magnesium with vitamin C and found that such a preparation seemed to localize at the site of the cancer. There were no unpleasant side effects. Instead, the average patient had a sense of well-being, became cheerful and active and had an increased appetite and an improved condition of the blood. Toxic symptoms such as vomiting and diarrhea disappeared. In some cases the tumor became so much smaller that it could be removed by operation.

The two physicians state their belief that such a treatment is infinitely preferable to giving drugs, even in the case of hopeless cancer. They say, "From our experience in hopeless cases we would like to stress that many patients are alive today simply because we resisted the temptation to give them the inevitable quarter grain of morphia. We would stress that no patient, as long as he is alive and breathing, should be abandoned and regarded as hopeless."

Results of Treatment Show Great Promise

The substance used by Dr. Meyer and described by him in an article written with G. G. Exner in *The Medical Press* for December 30, 1953, is called Complex ZA. This is the combination of zinc, magnesium and vitamin C. It is for intramuscular or intravenous injection.

Two hundred patients with advanced cancer who were treated with the vitamin-mineral complex showed significant improvement—relief from pain, prolongation of life with freedom from distressing symptoms. A few cases considered inoperable became operable. There was a return of appetite, increase in weight, and in leukemia improvement was immediate and "quite remarkable at times."

Meyer and Exner say they hope that their therapy,

[185]

by relieving pain in patients may overcome some of the dread most people have for cancer, which leads them to neglect important symptoms and to postpone the time for examination. We are told that such postponement is one reason for our high incidence of cancer. Geoffrey Murray in his book, *Frontiers of Healing* (Max Parrish, London, 1958) has much to say about Dr. Meyer's work. Mr. Murray gives one significant part of the complicated answer when he says, "Three out of every five surgeons practising today would lose their livings if cancer could be controlled by a pill or an injection which general practitioners, nurses, or even patients could administer to themselves, just as diabetics dose themselves with insulin."

Doesn't the theory add substance to the whole idea of the healthfulness of natural foods and natural vitamin and mineral supplements? Vitamin C does not function alone. Other substances are needed to assure its assimilation. Zinc and magesium are found in greatest abundance in other foods from those in which vitamin C is most abundant. They occur chiefly in seed products. Wheat bran (carefully removed when white flour is milled) is one of the richest sources of zinc. Wheat germ and brown rice are excellent sources of magnesium and zinc. Most Americans eat white flour products and refined rice. Can it be that a consistent deficiency in vitamin C, continuing day after day over a lifetime, combined with the consistent lack of certain minerals (perhaps zinc and magnesium are the most important) could be one of the basic causes of cancer?

We think that this is the stuff of real scientific

[186]

research. We think that Dr. Meyer's discoveries and the results of his treatment should have made banner headlines in every newspaper in the world. Here is a breakthrough; here is definite proof of the relationship of nutrition to cancer. Yet, Dr. Meyer's work has been steadfastly ignored. Think of the thousands of cancer patients who might have lived, or might have died painless and easy deaths had they known about Dr. Meyer's treatment. And think of the wasted four years during which laboratory research with full cooperation of government agencies might have come closer to solving the problem of cancer.

Geoffrey Murray in his book, *Frontiers of Healing,* has this to say about Dr. Meyer's work:

"The work of Dr. Meyer and his associates is so well documented and comes from men with such unassailable professional qualifications, that it is disquieting to find it has aroused so little attention from those engaged on research designed to bring relief to a suffering race. It may be that there are cogent reasons for ignoring it. If there are, then we should be told what these are, because now that their technique has been published, by reputable men in reputable publications, the hope has been aroused in the hearts of many under sentence of death that reprieve is possible. That hope may be false. To keep it alive if there is no justification for it would be inexcusably cruel. But acceptance or repudiation must be the result of adequate investigation. Instead, the new therapeutic agent and the results seemingly achieved by it are merely being ignored. Why?"

[187]

CHAPTER XIX

Is Insulin The Cancer Breakthrough?

A small-town American doctor and a group of Russian scientists have come up with independent evidence that insulin, the standard treatment for diabetes, may also be an effective anti-cancer agent. They share this theory with a New Jersey physician, and many of the German medical fraternity. Yet with the millions being spent yearly on cancer research, we know of no U.S. investigation into this promising lead.

One case of which we have learned is that of Mrs. Robert Tisdale, mother of two daughters, diagnosed as a victim of Hodgkin's Disease (cancer of the lymph glands) in 1958. Four operations to reduce the painful and distressingly persistent lumps which appeared

[188]

in the groin and neck area had seen Mrs. Tisdale slip closer to death. When still another operation was scheduled, she refused, and left the hospital over the protests of physicians who warned her that without surgery she would probably be dead in two weeks.

Literally Carried In

"I didn't know what I was going to do when I got home; I only knew that the operations hadn't helped, and I was determined not to have another," recalls Mrs. Tisdale. This attractive and vivacious lady describes her first visit to Dr. Samuel Beale, a Sandwich, Massachusetts, M.D. "A friend who knew how desperately ill I was took me to see Dr. Beale. I had to be literally carried into the office. He gave me my first shot of insulin that day in November, 1962. By Christmas I was driving my own car and doing my own housework. I haven't had a sick day since."

Mrs. Tisdale goes to the hospital for periodic checkups and blood tests to be certain that the disease is still under control. Doctors have come from many parts of New England to check her story and her charts. They find it difficult to believe they are dealing with the same person whose apparently hopeless condition is evidenced by the charts dated less than two years ago. There is no trace of Hodgkin's Disease in any of the current tests they do. "They tell me they don't understand it, but that they wouldn't miss an insulin shot if they were I, and I don't," Mrs. Tisdale said. "I give the injections to myself, one every other evening."

[189]

Dr. Beale's insulin-treated cases range from minor skin cancer to cancers of the eye and the breast. Records and pictorial slides show the progress they made. The need for surgery, he says, was eliminated in many of the cases and tumors unaccountably regressed and disappeared. "I have never claimed insulin as a cure for anything, but as an adjunct to accepted methods. This statement applies particularly to cancer, although sometimes insulin alone is all that is required."

Dr. Beale discovered insulin's regenerative action on abnormal tissue totally independent of any other research. In treating a near-gangrenous infection of the toe in a 63-year-old patient some thirty years ago, he found the patient slightly diabetic and began insulin injections. A remarkable improvement in the toe as well as the diabetes followed. The diabetes was soon controllable with diet alone. But when the insulin was stopped the toe changed for the worse. Dr. Beale suspected that the insulin had exerted a healing influence on the degenerating tissue of the toe. He began using small doses of insulin for healing and has continued using it on ulcers and other serious skin breaks from that time, with no dangerous side effects.

Dr. Beale did not realize then that the rationale for using insulin to treat cancer was gaining support. Scientists knew then that each cell contains a minute amount of insulin. Was this factor missing from malignant cells? Dr. Beale believes so, and he believes that this lack causes the cell to go haywire.

Magical Catalyst

Insulin, a natural product of the pancreas, cannot be chemically synthesized. The insulin used pharmaceutically is derived from animals. Professor Isaac Asimov has called it a catalyst "almost magical in its properties." (A catalyst is a substance which must be present to set off a chemical reaction, though the substance itself does not change during the reaction.) The reaction encouraged by insulin in the cells is oxidation, the burning of oxygen. This gives the cell its energy and promotes its proper function, says Dr. Beale. No other substance but insulin can do this job as nature intended, and that is why all normal cells are equipped with it, says Beale. He suggests that malignant cells short on insulin, or without it entirely, use sugar erratically, through undisciplined fermentation. He believes that insulin, restored to the cells through injections of small doses (2 to 3 units) will encourage malignant cells to revert to a normally regulated energy supply.

Critics have raised the question that if an insulin shortage of the cells is related to the development of cancer, all diebetics should be likely candidates for this disease (we know of no proof that this group is any more susceptible than others), and diabetics who have cancer should be relieved of the cancer when insulin is used. Dr. Beale answers that the exact cause of diabetes is not yet understood by medical men. Diabetes itself may be caused by the body's inability to use insulin properly, rather than any actual shortage of this hormone. Also, the effect of the minute

[191]

doses of insulin Dr. Beale prescribes is entirely different from that of the large doses used in treating diabetes. The doctor is very insistent on the necessity of limited doses of insulin in the treatment.

While Dr. Beale may be the American physician most experienced in using insulin to treat cancer, he is not the only one using it. Serge A. Koroljow, M.D., a New Jersey physician, reported on insulin for cancer in *Psychiatric Quarterly,* April, 1963. He is convinced, too, that somehow insulin can help to control the spread of cancer in some (not all) cases. Koroljow believes the insulin somehow interferes with the capacity of cancer cells to reproduce, or it might act to strengthen the normal cells which border the cancer so that they can resist invasion.

There are at least ten danger signs of cancer, not just the seven made so famous by the American Cancer Society. Here are three symptoms that are seldom mentioned: cancer patients are constipated, have a low urinary output, and have weak capillaries, according to Dr. Koroljow. This does not mean that all people who show these three symptoms have cancer, but they do indicate that an examination for cancer should be done.

Dr. Koroljow, a board certified psychiatrist, became involved with the diagnosis and treatment of cancer accidentally. But what was at first a casual interest developed into a serious research project into the basic mechanics of cancer.

In 1957, Dr. Koroljow, as a psychiatrist, happened to treat a lady of 53 for extreme depression. He saw

[192]

her first about six weeks before she had an operation for cancer of the cervix. He noted in his report, published in the *Psychiatric Quarterly* (April, 1962), that the operation showed hopeless cancer. The patient was put on pain-killing drugs. She still had the mental difficulties which had started about three years earlier.

No Signs of Malignancy

It was under these circumstances that Dr. Koroljow began a course of "ambulatory (sub-coma) insulin treatment" for her depression. By the end of the fourth week, "improvement, both in her mental and physical condition, took place. She became considerably less restless and agitated, and her depression almost completely disappeared. . . . But strangely enough, instead of continuing to lose weight, she gained two pounds, felt stronger physically, and her appetite improved. By the end of the fifth week, A. C. stopped taking all kinds of drugs and slept fairly well five to six hours a night. . . . Approximately one week after the course of insulin treatment was terminated, she was examined by her surgeon and he could not detect any signs of malignancy. A biopsy was done again, and it showed completely normal cellular morphology."

A second patient, M.C., a single woman aged 62, had similar results. This patient also had a cancer diagnosis. When she was told of it, the patient became depressed and attempted suicide. Again insulin treatment was begun. After nine weeks of treatment, M. C. had gained 17½ pounds, depression was gone and she

[193]

felt good. The swelling had rapidly diminished in size. After the 15th week the treatment was discontinued since all swelling and pain had disappeared. Four years later the patient was completely normal both physically and mentally. She had resumed her duties as a social worker.

These experiences kindled Dr. Koroljow's interest in the action of insulin against cancer. He had several other patients in whom the insulin treatment did not improve the cancer. Why did it work on some and not on others? In an effort to understand the anticancer activity of insulin fully, Dr. Koroljow kept extremely close records, full of minute detail, on the cancer patients he saw and treated. The records showed a consistent pattern of constipation, limited urine output and weak capillaries.

Constipation Relief—Cancer Improved

The degree of constipation was in direct ratio to the progress of the patient. When the patient seemed improved, he found that the constipation had been relieved. English physicians have long maintained that cancer is nourished by the constipated bowel. Koroljow concluded that unless the bowels could be brought to reasonably normal function, prognosis for the cancer patient was poor.

Cancer patients produce very little urine, says Koroljow, and what urine is produced is heavily concentrated. As the cancers improve, the urine flow improves. Dr. Koroljow prescribed diuretics to increase the urine flow. Even drug-induced urine output seemed

[194]

to improve the patients, at least in attitude and lessening of pain. The doctor used the diuretics in conjunction with insulin and sulfasuxadine. The sulfa was used to kill bacterial flora which he suspected might be feeding the cancer in constipated patients.

Finally Koroljow observed that the high and low periods, characteristic of many cancer patients, were reflected in the strength of their capillaries. A patient who had an uncomfortable period, and remarked finally that he felt better, invariably showed strong well-defined capillaries. The opposite was true when cancer patients complained of discomfort.

Dr. Koroljow tried various synthetic nutrients to improve the strength of the capillaries, but in spite of reported evidence for the value of particular vitamins in this area, only vitamin B_{12} brought results.

In attempting to correlate his observations Dr. Koroljow came up with this possible explanation. With constipation and urine retention, water is retained. The excess water dilates the capillaries until they burst. The liquid is absorbed by tissues. When the capillaries of the intestines collapse the intestinal tissues swell, and the swelling causes constipation.

What Does Insulin Do?

How does insulin fit into this picture? It conserves oxygen because it lowers blood sugar levels. With less sugar to be oxidized (burned), oxygen is allowed to accumulate in the blood and nourish the cells. Cancer cells are notably short of oxygen.

Insulin might also be a low-grade allergen which

[195]

attracts antibodies (protein) from feeding the cancer to fighting the insulin. If the body's war against insulin is sustained long enough, the cancer is deprived of the nourishment it needs and eventually it shrinks. This is the theory; there is no proof that it is true. Government work is now going on in investigating further the possibilities of insulin treatment for cancer.

Only time and further study will show the ultimate importance of Dr. Koroljow's observations. But we know already that a good diet, rich in fresh fruits and vegetables and as little processed as possible, is an excellent preventive against constipation. The B vitamins contained in brewer's yeast and desiccated liver are particularly valuable in handling this problem. Vitamin C works to maintain good kidney function, and vitamin A is an essential to the health of the mucous membranes in the urinary tract. Finally, vitamin C and the bioflavonoids are both vital to the strength of the capillaries. (Unfortunately Dr. Koroljow was not successful with vitamin therapy, perhaps because he used synthetics.)

In Germany It's Routine

We were surprised to learn from Dr. Koroljow that in Germany insulin is used routinely in the treatment of cancer. In Russia results have been demonstrated that make the outcome of accepted cancer treatments in the United States appear very pale indeed. One Russian report describes sixteen cancer patients treated with insulin. Four of the patients recovered completely; ten had temporary remission of three to six months, and

[196]

two showed no change. In Italy and Spain, as well as in South America, insulin is an orthodox part of cancer therapy, says Koroljow. In the United States, it is barely known.

The evidence currently available in recognized medical journals throughout the world is certainly not enough to seal the value of insulin as a sure cure for cancer. We all need to see much more work done on safety, optimal dosage and insulin's action on various types of cancer. The evidence would seem enough, however, to warrant serious consideration of insulin as a promising possibility in the cancer war. It can be used without interrupting orthodox treatments, if the attending physician prefers to do so. The National Cancer Institute, as well as non-government hospitals and universities whose laboratories receive public funds for cancer research, can hardly afford to postpone any longer a new look at insulin, this time as a cancer treatment.

[197]

CHAPTER XX

Starvation Treatment for Tumors

A cancer that can't grow is a cancer that won't kill. That is the basis for a new approach to fighting cancer now being explored by Dr. Albert B. Lorincz, professor of obstetrics and gynecology at the University of Chicago. Cancers that remain small are generally harmless and cause almost no discomfort. It is when a cancer grows and invades vital organs, displacing essential tissues, that it threatens life. Dr. Lorincz' strategy is to starve cancer cells into submission by withholding a protein element that is essential to their development.

A preliminary report in the *Nebraska State Medical Journal* (December, 1965) by Dr. Lorincz, along with Robert E. Kuttner, Ph.D., described this new concept in managing malignant disease. The theory is basically this: Any cell population undergoing rapid division and growth requires an enormous supply of protein to keep going. In fact, the demand for protein by malignant tumors is 1.3 to 11 times the level necessary for normal tissues. The doctors reasoned that the protein available to the malignant cells would be curtailed enough to hamper growth if an essential amino acid were lacking in the diet. The next problem faced by Dr. Lorincz: choose the right amino acid and devise a diet in which its appearance would be limited, yet nutritious enough to sustain the cancer patient.

Preliminary animal experiments by other researchers had shown that diets deficient in phenylalanine and lysine (both are amino acids) would inhibit the growth of liver cancer and breast cancer in mice. Further investigation disclosed that a low phenylalanine diet permits mice to maintain the weight, hemoglobin level and plasma proteins essential to life, while inhibiting tumor growth. In human adult females the minimum phenylalanine requirement is estimated between 420 and 620 milligrams a day. With another amino acid, tyrosine, present in sufficient amounts the phenylalanine requirement goes down to between 120 and 220 milligrams a day. A formula combining the proper amounts of tyrosine and phenylalanine was chosen as the experimental medication.

Selective Cell Starvation

Dr. Lorincz' treatment is essentially a process of selective cell starvation. He reasons that the cells that need phenylalanine the most (the rapidly dividing cancer cells) will suffer most from not having it. Experimental patients were put on a strict diet with limited

[199]

supplements of certain fruits, vegetables, cereals, fats and carbohydrates, all aimed at keeping phenylalanine down so that the total amount of this amino acid remained much lower than ordinary. Patients ate this way for four weeks, followed by three to five weeks of unrestricted food intake. Then the low phenylalanine diet began again for another 28-day period. During this time periodic blood samples and tissue specimens were obtained for analysis.

As is usual with such experimental procedure, only patients who were considered beyond the help of orthodox medical treatment were placed on the diet. It was gratifying to find that after weeks or months some of the cancer regressed and many of the patients were relieved of pain. Some of the patients were able to resume their normal activities.

One of the most striking cases concerns a woman who had been bedridden for a year, and in spite of all other treatments was so thoroughly riddled with cancer that her doctor called her "more cancer than person." She was kept alive only by repeated blood transfusions. After three months on the diet, and with no other treatments, she was up and walking. In time she was able to take her regular activities as a housewife and mother.

Condition: Grave and Unresponsive

In the *Nebraska Journal* Lorincz describes a 52-year-old woman suffering from Hodgkin's Disease (cancer of the lymph glands) since January, 1958. She was "extensively and exhaustively treated by radiation and drugs." As the disease got worse, more radical treatments, including nitrogen mustard gas, were administered periodically over the next five years. Still the disease worsened until December, 1962, when anemia became so acute that regular blood transfusions were begun. Over the next three years the patient fought fever, nausea, lack of appetite and progressive weight loss. Therapy of all types continued, along with drugs for pain.

When the phenylalanine diet was started in December, 1962, "the patient's condition was grave and unresponsive to all forms of conventional therapy." She was now in her seventh year of battling the disease. Her condition gradually improved and continued to do so with the phenylalanine restriction. For the first time in five years she showed a gain of weight and was also able to walk outside her home. The blood condition improved for the first time without a transfusion. "Her general feeling of well-being amazed all who knew her, and her attending physician reported a definite decrease in the bulk of the enlarged diseased pelvic nodes."

The results are encouraging but Dr. Lorincz firmly states that the treatment is not a cure for cancer. For one thing, the cancer remains under control only so long as the diet is in force. Patients who go off the diet for an appreciable period, even after a good initial result, see a return of the same symptoms as before, and doctors agree that there is a renewal of dangerous growth.

What the diet does offer to seriously ill cancer pa-

[201]

tients is the hope of shrinking cancers diagnosed as inoperable, to a size that permits their removal by surgery. This result was achieved in one patient judged to be beyond surgery. After five months on the diet, his cancer receded to a point where surgery proved possible and successful.

Patients on the diet complain that it is tasteless and monotonous. Nobody denies this, but efforts are being made to improve it both in flavor and texture. As the diet stands now it is barely palatable, admittedly difficult to prepare and expensive. Patients must stay with it strictly for the first four weeks, so they are hospitalized in the beginning to make sure.

Over the years there have been numerous cancer treatments based on diet, but none of them has been accepted by orthodox medicine in the United States. Physicians freely admit that the cancer operations they undertake are sometimes hopeless, and the drugs they employ have side-effects that are seriously dangerous, yet they shy away from trying diet as a treatment for cancer.

Dr. Lorincz frankly admits that his diet is still experimental, neither perfected nor completely proved. He wants more trial and more experimentation. Cancer patients and their families will be anxiously waiting to see if he gets any support. Will a promising treatment, free from side-effects and apparently successful, at least in some cases, attract the attention of enough cancer researchers to find out for sure if phenylalanine restriction is the chance for life cancer victims are praying for?

[202]

Same Approach to Leukemia

A very similar startling success has been recorded by a group of researchers based at the Wadley Institute of Molecular Medicine in Dallas, Texas.

The six doctors who reported on their new therapy in the *Journal of the American Medical Association* (Nov. 27, 1967) have taken what is fundamentally the same approach to leukemia. Their report also offers the first definite hope that we are aware of that a way to fight the metastatic spread of cancer may also have been found.

Here is the similarity: Dr. Lorincz found that tumor cells must have the amino acid, phenylalanine, or they will die. Healthy cells also require the same amino acid, but they are better able to adapt to a deprivation of it. So Dr. Lorincz has been using a nophenylalanine diet for a limited period of time—usually thirty days—in the course of which he has caused tumors to shrink appreciably as some of their cells died for lack of the amino acid, while the healthy cells of the body were able to get along without the amino acid for that length of time. It is his hope that repeated cycles of starvation and feeding of this particular amino acid will result eventually in complete regression of tumors, which is to say cure. And the Texas group, similarly, has discovered another amino acid—asparagine—that seems to be indispensable to tumor cells but to whose absence healthy cells can adapt.

Enzyme Destroys Asparagine

Their method of starving the malignant tissue, how-

[203]

ever, differs markedly. Instead of relying on a diet that would starve the person for this particular amino acid, they use an enzyme that they discovered in the blood of guinea pigs that specifically destroys asparagine. Called, therefore, L-asparaginase, this enzyme has been obtained thus far only from guinea pigs and one strain of bacteria and is in very short supply. The supply is so limited that the entire existing quantity can be used only for experimental work to try to gain further knowledge of just how effective or disappointing it may prove in wider trials aimed at combating cancer. If its success should be confirmed, then ways to synthetize the enzyme—which is also a protein substance composed of amino acids—will be sought and, there is little doubt, will be found.

Most encouraging, the Texas researchers who initiated this field of study reported not only the reduction of tumors of various lymph glands (a common form of leukemia) but also that they have been able to kill malignant cells that had already been disseminated throughout the lymphatic system. It is well known, of course, that the fact that cells break off from the primary tumor and spread either through the bloodstream or the lymphatics or both is one of the reasons that there are so few cures of cancer even through successful surgery. And if a way has now been found to destroy not only the cells of a tumor but also the free disseminated cells that would in time form other tumors in other locations, by starving them for asparagine, that is a giant step forward indeed.

One of the organizations that has been checking on

the pioneering work of Drs. Hill, Roberts, Loeb, Kahn, MacLellan and Hil in Texas, has been the Memorial Sloan-Kettering Cancer Center in New York. Results obtained there by a 10-man research team were reported to a meeting of the American Association of Hematology in Toronto, Ontario on December 4, 1967. The report was inconclusive.

Favorable Response in 50%

Dr. Herbert F. Oettgen said it may be many years yet until the true effectiveness of L-asparaginase will be known. He said that preliminary tests in 14 patients in New York did not attempt cures but were aimed at finding out whether human cancers would respond to the enzyme in the same way animal tumors do. There was a favorable response in eight of the 14 patients tested. However, Dr. Oettgen indicated that it is now virtually sure that not all types of cancer cells will respond to this particular form of therapy. Of the eight patients showing a favorable response, seven were suffering from the same type of acute leukemia. But among patients with a different type of the same disease, only one showed a favorable response while three others did not.

One of the big problems, therefore, is to determine specifically and precisely just which types of cancer cells can be treated by this particular enzyme.

A Control, Not a Cure

Another strong indication that has been found is that the enzyme cannot actually be expected to "cure" any-

[205]

one, although it may be quite successful as a continuing treatment. Among the eight patients reported by Dr. Oettgen as showing a favorable response, three showed a complete disappearance or remission of their leukemia which could have been considered a cure if it could have been sustained. However, the disease returned after nine weeks in one patient and after 11 weeks in a second, while only one patient has continued free of the disease for about six months.

This would indicate that, just like phenylalanine deprivation, destruction of asparagine in the system must be considered less as a potential cure for cancer than as potentially a more successful continuing treatment for the disease. In this respect, the comment of the Texas doctors in the AMA journal as to side-effects is highly significant. "When highly purified, L-asparaginase is apparently without acute toxicity; specifically no fever, mucous membrane lesions, bleeding tendency, alopecia, or jaundice was observed. No pulmonary changes were noted nor were any symptoms associated with the high blood-ammonia levels."

There are side-effects, but they are not nearly as dangerous nor as difficult to endure as the side-effects of radiation and chemical poisons, the commonly used therapies of today.

There is every reason to hope that the new field of research into the infinite metabolic roles of the amino acids will at the very least bring about a great improvement in effectiveness and a reduction in adverse consequences in the treatment of cancer.

CHAPTER XXI

Laetrile and a New Approach to the Cancer Problem

Among the many trails that have been followed by researchers seeking the cause, prevention and treatment of cancer is a fascinating one involving the nature of the first cell of a human being—that tiny center of life which divides into two cells. One of the theories which developed is called today by Howard H. Beard, Ph.D., the "trophoblastic theory of malignancy."

Dr. Beard bases his ideas on the original ideas of Dr. John Beard, (who is no relation to him)—professor of Embryology at the University of Edinburgh—"the only individual who was destined to solve the riddle of cancer" according to the present Dr. Beard. The embryologist discovered the nature of cancer, according to Dr. Beard, in 1902, and suggested the use of pancreatic enzymes in treating it. He published a book on the treatment of cancer in 1911.

[207]

Dr. Howard Beard, who lives and works in Texas, published a book in 1958 on this theory and treatment of cancer which is called *A New Approach to the Conquest of Cancer, Rheumatic and Heart Diseases* (Pageant Press, New York). Dr. Beard tells us that the earlier book formed the basis of treatment at the John Beard Research Institute in San Francisco. He later developed tests for cancer which have proved, he says, to be 95 per cent reliable. He tells us, further, that ten different groups of doctors in this country, in England, Italy, Belgium, Japan and the Philippines are using his ideas and his treatment for cancer.

Dr. Beard says, in the introduction to his book, "The conquest of cancer will only be accomplished by the cooperation of the public and the clinicians. The clinicians cannot treat cancer without documented proof of the effect of any new therapy of cancer and the public doesn't know the cancer story. It is hoped that if the layman gets bored with reading so many case histories, just let him put himself in that patient's shoes and then the story will be entirely different. The greatest mistake made today is that almost 100 per cent of the population believes that the other fellow will get cancer but he will never get it himself. Cancer is no respecter of persons; it can attack anyone at any time. Hence, the only way to convince the doctor and the public that the cancer problem is solved is to cite many case histories where recoveries have occurred under chymotrypsin and laetrile therapy."

These are the two substances used by Dr. Beard in treating cancer. He also has developed a test which, he says, will show the presence of malignancy long before it could be detected by biopsy; giving injections of laetrile, he claims, can prevent the discovered cancer or tendency to cancer from developing into malignancy.

Laetrile is a drug developed by Dr. Ernst T. Krebs that is extracted from the kernels of apricot seeds. It contains pangamic acid and strychnine in a special form that is said to be more deadly to the cancer cell while relatively less harmful to normal tissue.

Banned both by the FDA and the State of California, where it was originally made, it is not available anywhere in the United States. It is used experimentally by the McNaughton Foundation of Montreal, Canada, and Laetrile treatments are being administered to cancer patients in Mexico. There are hundreds of people who believe that Laetrile is responsible for their being alive today.

What Is the Theory?

As we understand it, the basis of the theory is this: a certain kind of cell produced in the pregnant female is the same kind of cell that becomes the cancer cell. It is simply a question of where the cells develop, says Dr. Beard. Pregnancy and malignancy are analogous— that is, the same, in some aspects. Pregnancy is physiological and sexual. Malignancy is asexual and, from the clinical point of view, pathological or diseased. "The development of a malignant tumor is simply an attempt of the asexual life to take over the sexual life of the individual," states Dr. Beard.

[209]

To put it another way, you might say that a cancerous cell is a cell that might have developed into a child. Instead, it is found in another part of the body, but it has the ability to divide and reproduce rapidly, as we know cancer cells do.

These potentially dangerous cells are controlled in the healthy individual by an enzyme, chymotrypsin, which, says Dr. Beard, prevents cancer just as insulin prevents diabetes. Insulin is, of course, a hormone, and chymotrypsin is an enzyme.

It seems reasonable, then, that if one could predict the development of cancer in an individual, he could administer the enzyme mentioned above and prevent the cancer from developing, just as insulin prevents diabetic symptoms in persons to whom it is administered. And Dr. Beard tells us that he has developed such a test. In this test, which Dr. Beard calls the Anthrone test, a certain substance is revealed which is present only in the urine of pregnant women and those who have a malignant or cancerous condition. Its amount is directly proportional to the degree of malignancy present.

The test is said to have shown an amazing degree of accuracy. It will not work in the case of pregnant women, women recently delivered of babies, women who have a certain kind of mole, in cases of male or female acromegaly (a disease of the pituitary gland), in uncontrolled diabetes or in advanced liver disease. Aside from these exceptions, the test is practically 100 per cent certain, according to Dr. Beard.

The center portion of Dr. Beard's book is devoted

[210]

to about 60 pages of case histories of cancer patients treated with Laetrile. Dr. Beard believes that "cancer cures" claimed by orthodox medicine for x-ray or surgery cases are not "cures" at all. He says that the cancer patient suffers from a lack of the enzyme, chymotrypsin. "Once a cancer patient has developed a tumor, this patient is suffering from a chymotrypsin deficiency and this patient will always be a chymotrypsin deficient patient regardless of treatment or no treatment. A tumor may show up as long as 60 years after the patient has been pronounced cured."

Basic Nature of the Therapy

Our interest in Dr. Beard's work stems partly from the very basic nature of the theory—relating cancer to the beginning of life, as well as his description of cancer as a deficiency disease. We were extremely interested in his test for potential cancer and we think such a test holds very great promise for conquering cancer, if indeed it will indicate the presence of malignancy early in the game when steps can be taken to reverse the state.

Finally, we were interested in Dr. Beard's story because, throughout his entire career, orthodox medicine has turned a stony ear to what he has to say. It does not recognize Dr. Beard's work with even so much as a nod. Dr. Beard has taught at several universities— Western Reserve, Louisiana State, Chicago Medical School. His employment has been hazardous, because it is dangerous, these days, to talk of your own work in cancer treatment.

[211]

We say of his book, his treatment and his test for cancer, just what we have said of Krebiozen, Mucorhicin and the Gerson treatment, we do not know whether or not he can do what he says he can do. His evidence sounds impressive and impelling. We are not cancer experts.

We believe it is the job of the experts—chiefly the National Cancer Institute, a government department established to deal with matters like this—to test any such claims and such treatments—to test them fairly, objectively, and with the greatest good will. We, who pay the taxes, assume that the National Cancer Institute is there to find the answer to this terrible disease. They dare not—*they simply dare not*—neglect or slight or damn with faint praise any cancer treatment or test that shows promise, let alone one where the evidence is as convincing as Dr. Beard's. We urge readers to demand a congressional investigation which will bring to light all such work done in all parts of the country along with an explanation from our government bureaus as to why they persist in repressing, discouraging and attacking such work. Can it be, as Dr. Beard says flatly, that the medical profession does not want to find a cure for cancer?

Part Four:

NUTRITION AND THE
AVOIDANCE OF CANCER

CHAPTER XXII

Cancer and Nutrition

"If man would keep himself fit instead of fat, the chances are that cancer would be less of a menace to the human race than it is. There is evidence from animal experiments that caloric restriction reduces the incidence of several types of tumors; there is statistical evidence, from various insurance companies, that overweight persons have a distinctly greater tendency for developing cancer."

These words are from *The Challenge of Cancer,* published by the National Cancer Institute, a department of the Public Health Service. So even the most conservative sources of information recognize that cancer is definitely related to diet. Yet the average M.D., asked if cancer has anything to do with diet, will tell you that such ideas are the disproved notions of food faddists and cranks.

Do we have any background for saying that diet

[215]

influences the incidence of cancer? There is much material available on this subject. As you read on in this book, you will be amazed.

More than a decade ago we became convinced there is a relationship between what you eat or don't eat, and whether or not you develop cancer. Let us begin with what we have known since 1957, and then present the mass of evidence that has accumulated since.

A Spanish medical magazine, *Revista Clinica Espanola* for October 15, 1956, describes an experiment in which a hundred and twenty people living in a residential home for the aged were divided into two groups, an experimental group and a control group. The experimental group received a diet amounting to 2300 calories on alternate days. On the other days, they received only about a quart of milk and a pound of fresh fruit. The control group received the 2300 calorie diet every day.

At the end of three years the number of days in which persons in either group had reported to the hospital department of the home was twice as great for persons in the control group as for those who got a so-called starvation diet every other day. The incidence of heart and blood vessel disease, cancer and bronchitis was twice as high in those in the control group. The results of the experiment showed, the authors feel, that the hunger diet on alternate days maintains a feeling of well-being in the elderly and prolongs the health and life span. Chalk up point one for a sensible, moderate diet, high in natural foods.

As long ago as 1946, D. H. Copeland W. D. Salmon

at the Alabama Polytechnic Institute published in the *American Journal of Pathology* for September, 1946, the results of their experiments with rats in which they showed that a deficiency in just one of the B vitamins, choline, resulted in an incidence of 58 per cent cancer in laboratory rats, whereas the second group of rats, fed exactly the same diet, with added choline, had no cancers at all.

In 1950 E. R. Jaffe, R. W. Wisser and E. P. Benditt reported in the *American Journal of Pathology* for September, 1950, that rats given high amounts of choline and two of the amino acids (forms of protein), methionine and cystine, had far less cirrhosis of the liver than those which received less. This disease is closely related to cancer of the liver.

The Denver Post for December 12, 1954, told of the findings of Dr. Clarence G. Salsbury, Arizona's Public Health Commissioner, who found that the Navajo Indians, ravaged by disease for centuries, were very infrequently victims of cancer. Of 60,000 hospital admissions among Navajos, only 208 cancer cases had ever been seen. Among 118 female cases only three breast cancers had ever been recorded. "The typical primitive Navajo diet does not include highly refined foods," Salsbury said. "It consists mainly of meat, corn, squash, some fruits and nuts, herbs, native tea and 'squaw bread'—a type of crisp panbread. That simple diet may be the key to the comparative lack of cancer. But just why or how we don't yet know."

Nutrition Reviews for March, 1956, reviewed the subject of overweight and cancer and showed that re-

[217]

stricting the diets of laboratory animals "markedly delayed" the appearance of both spontaneous and experimentally induced cancers.

An article by Associated Press Science Editor, Howard Blakeslee, tells of the theory of Dr. F. E. Chidester, author of a book, *Nutrition and Glands in Relation to Cancer*. Dr. Chidester believes that in the early stages of vitamin deficiency the human glands are overactive. This extra activity causes the body to lose enormous amounts of calcium, iodine and iron and, he claims, leads to goiter, anemia, diabetes, nerve degeneration, rickets, ulcers and so forth. In the later stages of vitamin deficiency, when the glands have become exhausted, a form of fat accumulates which leads to gallstones, cataracts, hardening of the arteries and the most malignant cancers. Dr. Chidester says vitamins are extremely important for keeping the glands working properly. He says that vitamins A, B and E have been tested in experimental cancers of animals with good results and that they have also been beneficial in some cases of human cancer.

Dr. W. C. Hueper of the National Cancer Institute, the gentleman who speaks so forcefully against chemicals in foods as possible cancer-causers, said that some dietary factors that affected the incidence of cancer were well established, according to an article in the *Milwaukee Journal* for October 11, 1956. Obesity is one. The amount of protein in the diet appears to be another, since liver cancer is much more common in nations in Asia and Africa where there is little protein in the diet. There are many substances added to our

[218]

food today which may be found some day soon to be cancer-causers, he said. The finding of gastrointestinal cancers mostly at sites where the stomach or intestines narrow, slowing the passage of food so that it is in contact longer there, was additional evidence that what we eat might influence the production of cancers. He predicted that, when more is learned about dietary factors in cancer, the disease would be controlled.

Seymour J. Kreshover, D.D.S. and John J. Salley, D.D.S., writing in the *Journal of the American Dental Association* for April, 1957, tell us that deficiency in vitamins A and B are definitely known to be responsible for some mouth cancers. Cancer of the female reproductive organs can result from lack of vitamin A—in many cases caused by faulty absorption of the vitamin due to lack of hydrochloric acid in the stomach.

The book *Cancer, New Approaches, New Hope* by Boris Sokoloff (published by Devin Adair, New York, N. Y.) contains a stimulating chapter on nutrition in relation to cancer. Dr. Sokoloff relates experiments in which cancer was prevented in laboratory animals by giving them brewer's yeast and desiccated liver at the same time that a substance known to cause cancer was given. He also tells us that other laboratory experiments showed clearly that diets high in carbohydrates increase cancer incidence, while adding to the protein content of the diet reduces the number of cancers, in *every instance*. He tells us that animals kept on "purified" diets are more susceptible to cancer than those kept on a natural diet. A certain enough warning against refined foods, don't you think? Dr. Sokoloff

[219]

also tells us that normal tissue begins to change very decidedly before a cancer growth is detected. "The intercellular substance which binds together the cells, undergoes peculiar changes. . . . The cells are less adhesive each to the other, more free to move and to live independently." We know that vitamin C is responsible for the health of the intercellular substance. And this leads us to:

The theory of Dr. W. J. McCormick of Toronto, Canada, published in *Archives of Pediatrics* for October, 1954. Dr. McCormick believes that tissue may become susceptible to cancer through a breakdown of the intercellular cement due to vitamin C deficiency.

A high consumption of salt may be responsible for a predisposition to cancer. There is a low incidence of the disease among peoples who use little salt. It is true that too much salt in the diet may produce a mineral imbalance, since the sodium of table salt is the chemical enemy of potassium—a mineral in which we are likely to be deficient.

Here are some further facts to be taken into account. *Newsweek* for November 28, 1949, told of experiments performed at the Medical Research Department of the University of Toronto. For six weeks researchers fed one group of rats on alcohol instead of drinking water and another group of rats the same amount of sugar as that contained in the alcohol. Both sets of rats lost their appetite for food containing choline, that most important B vitamin which protects the liver from harm. Another indication of the deadly nature of sugar. Isn't it pathetic to think of all the fine, earnest Ameri-

[220]

can mothers, horrified at the thought of giving alcohol to their children, but who regularly feed them a substance that is just as harmful from the point of view of good health—white sugar! The liver, as we know, is one of the most important organs in the body and its health is essential for preventing cancer.

Another link in the chain tying cancer to poor nutrition comes from an article in *Science* for April 12, 1946, by Drs. J. Ernest Ayre and W. A. G. Bauld of the Royal Victoria Hospital and McGill University, Montreal. These researchers believe that the lack of a B vitamin, thiamin, may be the first link in a chain leading by way of the liver and female hormones to cancer of the uterus. "If tests show a dangerous precancerous linkage between low vitamin and high female hormone concentration, prevention of cancer might be possible through corrective treatment."

The doctors suggest that the vitamin lack might begin to operate by damaging the liver. This damage might be slight, so slight that it could not be perceived by any known tests of liver function. But even so, it might be enough to keep the liver from inactivating female hormone, which is one of its functions. This material might, then, accumulate in the body and cause cancer of the uterus.

Studies of 23 patients as well as various laboratory experiments give, say the scientists, "excellent circumstantial evidence that the nutritional deficiency may have been a primary factor leading to the malignancy." Has your cancer society or your doctor ever told you of such a theory? And if not, why not? The

[221]

B vitamins are practically non-existent for many modern women, in whose diets coffee, soft drinks, bakery products, packaged desserts and sweets play a big part. Doesn't it seem likely that present-day food habits have a lot to do with cancer of the uterus, in the light of this theory?

Cancer and Food Chemicals

Finally, there can be no consideration of food in relation to cancer that does not take into account the many, many chemicals in today's food.

In *Prevention of Chronic Illnesses,* prepared by the Commission on Chronic Illnesses and published by Harvard University Press, Cambridge, Massachusetts, 1957, we were astonished to find in the chapter on cancer a three page list, in small type, of various substances *known to cause cancer.* Here are some of them: Benzene, coal tar, asphalt, creosote oil, lubricating oils, petroleum products, fuel oils, soot, arsenic, chromates, nickel, asbestos, estrogens, carbon tetrachloride, chloroform, DDT, tannic acid, dulcin (a synthetic sweetner), diethylene glycol (used in tobacco), coal oil, waxes and oils made from coal, certain dyes, cellophane, polyethylene. The list goes on and on.

In some cases the substance is well known as a cause of cancer in human beings. Such things as arsenic and petroleum products fall in this category. Other substances have been found to induce cancer in laboratory animals—dulcin (the artificial sweetner whose use in food is now forbidden, incidentally), estrogens (hormones), DDT, dyes.

[222]

Which of these might contaminate food? Arsenic is a widely used insecticide; of course DDT is, too. Synthetic hormones are now being used in meat animals, either injected or fed to them. Dyes occur in just about every processed food you buy. Nickel and chrome may contaminate food from metal containers. Carbon tetrachloride until recently banned was a grain fumigant (how much of it remains in the grain?). Tannic acid, which gives rats cancer of the liver, exists naturally in tea and coffee. Thiourea is a preservative used on citrus fruit. (How much of it is present in the orange juice you squeezed today?)

Polyethylene and cellophane are used in wrapping food. Under certain conditions they cause cancer in animals.

Dr. W. C. Hueper, a leading authority in the field of cancer, now retired from the National Cancer Institute, said that "the actual or possible existence of cancer hazards related to carcinogens (cancer-causing substances) in foodstuffs poses a serious public health problem, since the daily and lifelong exposure to such agents would represent one of the most important of the various potential sources of contact with environmental carcinogens for the population at large, acting on both the healthy and the sick, the metabolically normal and the abnormal alike."

Some twenty different categories of food additives were listed by Dr. Hueper who said that we simply do not know whether or not any given one of these may cause cancer (let alone know what the effect would be of getting a little of each of them every day—some-

[223]

thing which laboratory animals have never been subjected to). Some of these additives are: antioxidants (used to keep fatty foods from turning rancid on the shelf), synthetic sweeteners (saccharin is the best known—new ones appear frequently,) preservatives and sterilizing agents, shortenings (especially hydrogenated shortenings—the thick white ones).

What are the chances of testing all these chemicals now being used in food? There are probably close to a thousand now in use. It is said that, under present conditions, it would take 25 years to test by modern scientific techniques *just the dyes* that are being used at present in foods!

Dr. William E. Smith of Englewood, New Jersey, has said, in reference to stilbestrol (the hormone used to fatten meat animals), that marketed poultry has contained per bird up to 342,000 times the amount of the hormone which sufficed, as a daily dose, to induce cancer in mice. A cancer-causing dye formerly used in foods did not induce cancer in well-fed test animals, but would bring cancer in animals on less adequate diets. Can the manufacturer who puts this sort of dye in his product follow every customer out of the store to make certain he eats a nutritious diet so that the dye will not harm him?

Chemicals in food are there to make greater profit for the food processor. They serve no other purpose. They do not improve the food in any way for the consumer. But the consumer must pay (and how many pay with their lives?) for the extra profit made by using a preservative that prolongs the "shelf-life" of the product, by using dye that gives the product brighter color than that of a competitive product, by using a synthetic fat in place of a natural one and thus cutting costs, by using insecticides and fumigants and thus cutting down on losses. And so forth.

Avoid as much as you are able foods to which chemicals have been added. Do not buy processed foods, ever. Use fresh foods. These, too, have their share of poisons. The best possible diet and food supplements (especially vitamin C) will do much to protect you from harm. From cancer, too? We cannot be certain, but it seems likely. Many chemical poisons act by destroying some vitamin, mineral or enzyme in your body. If your diet supplies these in even larger quantities than you need, this alone constitutes some protection.

CHAPTER XXIII

B Vitamins Against Cancer

The treatment for cancer developed by Dr. Max B. Gerson is described in an official statement of the American Cancer Society as being "essentially that of diet. The principal ingredients stressed are liver, vitamins and fresh vegetables and fruit juices." The statement concludes that the cancer society "had found no acceptable evidence that treatment with the Gerson method results in any objective benefit. . . ."

We should like to call the attention of the cancer society to a recent paper by Dr. H. F. Kraybill, Ph.D., of the National Cancer Institute. Published in *Clinical Pharmacology and Therapeutics* (4,1, January-February, 1963) this paper coming from our top agency involved in cancer research has marshalled considerable evidence that nutritional treatment is of value both preventively and therapeutically, and that there

[226]

may be a great deal more to Dr. Gerson's theories than was thought possible ten years ago, when the cancer experts were laughing at him.

What is the Gerson theory? It was best stated by Dr. Gerson himself in his book *A Cancer Therapy*. "Cancer is not a single cellular problem; it is an accumulation of numerous damaging factors combined in deteriorating the whole metabolism, after the liver has been progressively impaired in its function. Therefore, one has to separate two basic components in cancer: a general one and a local one. The general component is mostly a very slow, progressing, imperceptible symptom caused by poisoning of the liver and simultaneously an impairment of the whole intestinal tract, later producing appearances of vitally important consequences all over the body."

The Liver Is the Key

In other words, it is the liver and its health that Dr. Gerson considers the core of the body's ability to resist cancer, and it is the malfunctioning of the liver that he believes is responsible for the weakening of the body's defenses and the ability of cancer to take hold. He states that "the damage is done by a permanent daily poisoning brought about by our modern civilization. This starts with the soil which is denaturalized by artificial fertilizers and depletion, thus gradually reducing the top soil. In addition, the soil is poisoned by sprays with DDT and other poisons. As a consequence, our nutrition is damaged. . . . Furthermore, the food

[227]

substances are damaged as they are refined, bottled, bleached, powdered, frozen, smoked, salted, canned and colored with artificial coloring. Carrots are sold in cellophane bags after having been treated for better preservation. Other foods contain damaging preservatives; finally, cattle and chickens are fed or injected with stilbestrol to accumulate more weight and be quickly ready for market."

Although the Sloan-Kettering Foundation has just begun to establish the fact that in a truly healthy person there is a cancer immunity and even the implantation of living, active cancer cells will quickly be overcome, this was something that Dr. Gerson knew and published in his book seven years ago. He believed that the source of immunity was a healthfully functioning digestive tract, particularly the liver. And his diet was directed toward cleansing the liver of accumulated poisons and building its health through a proper selection of nutrients.

Even though Gerson was called "one of the most eminent medical geniuses of the history of medicine" by the eminent physician Dr. Schweitzer, most of the medical profession, at least in the United States, considers that Gerson has been discredited. Yet if we are to judge by Dr. Kraybill's paper, some of today's cancer investigators may be engaged in rediscovering, slowly, methodically and painfully, just what Dr. Gerson was trying to tell them if they would only have listened.

Here are some of the discoveries that Dr. Kraybill has gathered together into his truly impressive paper:

[228]

Vitamin Value Documented

"Yeast is particularly effective (for the prevention of liver cancer) since the level of 15 per cent of it is almost completely protective, and any high quality protein diet and B vitamins, especially B2, are defensive mechanisms in inhibiting formation of such neoplasms."

"According to Cramer, certain precancerous lesions of the gastric mucosa such as gastric polyps, atrophic gastric ulcer and chronic atrophic gastritis have been attributed to deficiencies in vitamin A, riboflavin, and nicotinic acid. These lesions may advance into neoplasia in the presence of a carcinogen."

In the next paragraph, it is pointed out that it was necessary to deplete an experimental diet of thiamin and riboflavin in order to induce brain tumors with a chemical carcinogen.

"Perhaps the most interesting observations are those of Japanese and American investigators on liver neoplasia in which riboflavin-rich diets inhibited tumor formation. This preponderance of evidence on hepatomas associated with low B vitamin diets can probably account for the high tumor incidence among the Bantus and certain Asiatic groups.

"Hepatic tumors have also been reported to occur in rats when a choline-deficient diet was administered to a strain of rats having a high choline requirement. In general, the injury of liver cells resulting from a nutrient deficiency may impair normal growth of cells, and carcinogens may then readily induce hepatomatous nodules."

[229]

It will be noted that the nutrients pointed out by Dr. Kraybill as having a cancer-preventive effect are all foods that are directly concerned with the health of the liver. Thiamin, riboflavin and choline are all used principally in the liver, both for digestive functions and detoxification of the blood. When they are deficient, not only can the liver not function properly but it also deteriorates. Yeast, of course, is one of our most potent sources of the B complex vitamins. And it may also be presumed that there are other, still undiscovered food elements that are also necessary to liver health and may be deficient in many diets. That is perhaps why Dr. Gerson found that he got his best results by directly feeding raw liver, containing all known and unknown necessary liver nutrients, to his patients.

Additives Incriminated

When it comes to identifying those elements in food that may or may not be responsible for causing cancer, Dr. Kraybill again sounds remarkably like Dr. Gerson. He points out that "A consideration of food intake in carcinogenesis is not restricted to nutrition per se but must also include additives, contaminants, or processing degradation products which may play a more important role in tumor induction." And he then goes right down the list from heated or processed fats to spices, plastics, petroleum by-products and food colors and flavor additives as established or probable causes of cancer. These are all materials known to have toxic effects on the liver, and they are all materials that Dr.

[230]

Gerson attempted to keep out of the diets of his patients.

Dr. Kraybill cites 75 references, no less, all the authors of which have worked, established and published these facts for which Dr. Gerson only ten years ago was being called a quack and a faddist.

We find it especially interesting that while Dr. Kraybill does not cite Dr. Gerson and nowhere refers to the Gerson conclusion that the liver is the key organ in the body's resistance to cancer, just about all of his material deals with food elements that have a direct connection with liver health. The pesticides, food preservatives and colors, and the heated fats that occur in cooking all have their toxic effects on the liver and quite conceivably, may gradually diminish the body's resistance to cancer in this manner.

Certainly the 75 studies on which Dr. Kraybill based his paper as well as the pioneering work of Dr. Max Gerson give us every reason to believe that if we can keep our livers in good health, we are greatly improving our chances of being able to resist and overcome any incipient cancer. It is our belief that the very best food for liver health is liver itself. Liver, particularly when it has not been altered in any way by cooking, obviously would contain all those nutrient elements that are essential to liver function. These include a rich supply of the B complex vitamins, and several extremely important mineral elements such as phosphorus and magnesium. In desiccated liver, which is vacuum dried at comparatively low temperatures, all these elements are retained fully. And this is why desiccated liver is

[231]

one of the most valuable food supplements that can be included regularly in anybody's diet.

Yet when you get right down to it, the liver has so many functions in relation to health, from digestion to purification of the blood stream and addition to the blood of various food elements as they are required, that there is no nutrient that does not have some importance to the living, functioning liver. Brewer's yeast, a rich source of vitamin B and high grade protein, is certainly of enormous value. So are the A and D vitamins and there is recent evidence that the antioxidant functions of vitamins C and E are equally important.

Professor Otto Warburg

One of the world's great authorities on human physiology and particularly on the physiological development and effects of cancer is Professor Dr. Otto Warburg. Dr. Warburg, a Nobel Prize winner, is also director of the Max Planck Institute for Cell Physiology in Berlin, a world renowned institution. And it was no less an authority than Dr. Warburg who stated positively, in July, 1966, that some of the basic constituents of brewer's yeast and desiccated liver are precisely what each of us needs to give us the best possible chance of avoiding cancer throughout our lives.

The constituents named by Dr. Warburg are three of the B vitamins: riboflavin (vitamin B_{12}), niacin (vitamin B_3), and pantothenic acid.

Nor was it any casual statement about them that Dr. Warburg made, but rather it was presented as a scientific statement of key importance at a meeting in

Lindau, Germany, of the Nobel Prize recipients for 1966. Dr. Warburg's address was titled "Concerning the Ultimate Cause and the Contributing Causes of Cancer."

As Dr. Warburg explained the metabolic mechanics involved, although there are hundreds, perhaps thousands of secondary causes that stimulate and induce cancer, in the final analysis they are all reduced to a single primary cause.

Because of some harmful chemical stimulation, or radiation, or a weakness or error in the metabolism, a particular tissue becomes starved for oxygen. This can be because it is not receiving sufficient oxygen or because the enzyme system that permits the tissue to use oxygen has been damaged.

As little as a 35 per cent reduction in the oxygen available to the cell, according to Dr. Warburg, causes the cell in its efforts to stay alive to make a fundamental metabolic switch. It gives up attempting to derive its energy from the oxidation (or burning) of food and instead turns to securing energy by fermenting sugar, a process that requires no oxygen.

Respiratory Enzymes

Where do the B vitamins come in? The three named by Dr. Warburg—riboflavin, niacin and pantothenic acid—all act within our bodies as co-enzymes that are essential to the production and full activity of the respiratory enzymes within the individual cells. In other words, according to this scientist, a basic reason for the formation of a cancerous tumor may well be

[233]

that the particular tissues where the tumor forms lack one or another of these B vitamins and thus are unable to breathe properly. On the other hand, Dr. Warburg believes so firmly that these same vitamins in sufficient supply will activate and reinforce the necessary enzyme systems and thus prevent cancer, that he went so far as to suggest that following surgery for cancer, these vitamins would prevent the spread or recurrence of the fatal disease. The statement was not based on any kind of experimental evidence but was rather theoretical, depending on Dr. Warburg's long experience and enormous knowledge of the subject and coming from him as a suggestion for further investigation by other, younger top scientists. As brilliant a scientist as Dr. Warburg is, we would not go so far without clinical proof as to endorse his theoretical conclusion that the B vitamins in brewer's yeast would have an actual curative effect. When it comes to prevention, however, it is a different matter. There, there is plenty of evidence of a strong preventive effect that has unfortunately been ignored for the most part by the cancer establishment.

Evidence of Prevention

Fifteen years ago a fascinating and important experiment that took place at the Sloan-Kettering Foundation was reported. It was an investigation of cancer of the liver, a site of cancer that occurs so much more frequently in Japan, Korea and other Oriental countries than it does in the Occident that the difference is surely significant. (It is well known, of course, that the Oriental diet, consisting largely of polished rice, is deficient in the B-complex vitamins, particularly riboflavin.) Looking for a possible connection, a Japanese scientist, Dr. Kanematsu Sugiura, investigated liver cancer in laboratory rats. He fed the rats on a diet of polished rice to which, in order to speed up the study, he added a known cancer-causing substance called Butter Yellow, now prohibited but once used as a food dye to color oleomargarine. The rice and Butter Yellow mixture proved able to produce liver cancer in rats in 150 days' time.

Following this demonstration, Sugiura then took a new supply of rats and divided them into three groups, adding a fourth control group of 50. The control group was again fed a diet of rice and Butter Yellow. But of the other three groups, one was given the same diet with three per cent brewer's yeast added, the second had six per cent brewer's yeast, and the third 15 per cent.

In 150 days' time, all 50 animals in the control group receiving no yeast had developed cancer of the liver. All the other rats receiving various amounts of brewer's yeast in addition to the cancer-producing diet had smooth, normal livers. However, of those who received only three per cent brewer's yeast, 70 per cent later developed cancer nodules on their livers, and 30 per cent of the six per cent group developed some cancer nodules, though they were fewer.

None of the rats receiving 15 per cent brewer's yeast developed any sign of liver cancer.

For the final step in his experiments, Dr. Sugiura

[235]

induced liver cancer in a group of rats and then experimented to see whether feeding them brewer's yeast would have a curative effect as well. The results were not absolute. Out of 25 rats in whom liver tumors had been induced, feeding a diet of 15 per cent brewer's yeast for 250 days apparently wiped out the disease in 21 of them, but it did not help the other four.

"These dietary influences may prove to play a very large part in the causation, prevention and treatment of human cancer," stated Dr. Sugiura in an article in the *Journal of Nutrition* in 1951.

Desiccated Liver

So far as we know, there was only one single cancer experimenter and that one a man well outside the cancer establishment, without a single subsidy from any governmental or research organization, who followed up the Sugiura experiments. That man was Boris Sokoloff, M.D., who checked on the Sugiura experiments independently and confirmed that they really worked as described. Dr. Sokoloff also found that desiccated liver—as rich in the B vitamins as brewer's yeast—had an equally strong cancer preventive effect.

He then went on to try to isolate the particular element present in both yeast and liver that might be responsible for the effect. He found that riboflavin, alone, would effect a three per cent reduction in the incidence of cancer. Other single vitamins of the B group had no noticeable effect. Apparently it did not occur to Dr. Sokoloff—or perhaps he lacked the funds—to try various B vitamins in combination. If we are to

[236]

judge by Dr. Warburg's authoritative statement, a combination of the three B vitamins, riboflavin, niacin, and pantothenic acid, might have proven just as effective as whole brewer's yeast and whole desiccated liver.

Dr. Sokoloff published his confirmation of the Sugiura experiment in 1953. We have searched *Index Medicus,* the publication of the National Library of Medicine that lists all published medical articles within a given period, looking for any kind of follow-up on the enormously exciting and hopeful researches we have just described. It seems obvious to us that the next step was for a committee of experts to go to Japan or some other region where the incidence of liver cancer is high, and see whether a diet rich in brewer's yeast, desiccated liver or any other supplement that is rich in the B complex vitamins would have the same effect on a group of human beings. This, after all, is what is really important and what the world really wants to know.

To the best of our knowledge, no such study has ever been made.

Now, thirteen years later, it has remained for an aging expert in the field to use the weight of his scientific reputation to remind a group of winners of the Nobel Prize that he believes the B complex vitamins do have this protective effect and that it remains for them to conduct the studies that will either confirm or refute his beliefs.

How does brewer's yeast stack up against other foods as a source of B vitamins? Using riboflavin as a typical

[237]

example, here is a standard comparison from government figures:

Food	Mg. Per 100 Grams
Brewer's yeast	2,500 to 4,700
Lean pork	200
Dried Lima Beans	750 to 800
Liver	1,800 to 2,200
Kidney	1,700 to 2,200

The relationship is very much the same throughout the entire range of the B-complex vitamins. Milligram for milligram, brewer's yeast is the richest known source of the B vitamins, followed closely by desiccated liver. Desiccated liver is whole liver, air dried at temperatures low enough to avoid the loss of the food's precious nutrients while the water it contains is being slowly evaporated. The yeast is a plant—the smallest of all known plants—a single yeast being about the size of a red corpuscle in the human blood.

When you buy brewer's yeast as a food supplement, however, the yeast plants are no longer alive. Like desiccated liver, they are dried at very low temperatures to preserve the full nutritional values. This drying process kills the plants, which are then pulverized and given additional processing to remove a strong bitter taste that is native to yeast.

This natural source of a very rich supply of the B complex vitamins is believed by Dr. Otto Warburg to be the most valuable element you could add to your diet in order to keep your tissues in such a condition of health as to greatly improve your chances of avoiding cancer throughout life.

[238]

B Vitamins Fight Cancer of the Cervix

In spite of the efficacy of the Pap test, which greatly enhances the rate of detection of uterine cancer, this type of malignancy is the third ranking cause of cancer death among American women, and according to *Research Reports on Health Topics* published by Congressional Quarterly (1967) will devastate the lives of 14,000 women this year. Why?

Could it be because, as a nation, we are estrogen-happy and thiamin-deficient? Over 20 years ago, two research scientists made some penetrating studies at McGill University in Canada which accent the fact that "errors of diet leading to persistent or intermittent deficiency of such elements as thiamin might cause a persistent estrogenic growth stimulation over a period of years which, acting on a *'Locus minoris resistentiae'* (point of least resistance) such as an erosion, ultimately produces a malignant neoplasm."

Let's take a searching look at the report by J. Ernest Ayre and W. A. G. Bauld of the Gyne-cytology Laboratory, Royal Victoria Hospital, McGill University, Montreal published in *Science* (April 12, 1946).

During the course of making routine cytological studies on patients who were gynecological bleeders, Dr. Ayre and Dr. Bauld encountered three cases in whom similar cytology findings prompted further investigation. They all showed precancerous changes. All were bleeding excessively and all showed abnormally high estrogen levels in the cytology smears as well as thiamin *deficiency.*

[239]

"It has long been known, that certain coal tar products produce cancer with greater certainty than any other known chemical or physical irritant. The chemical structure of the responsible substance has been found to be similar to that of some of the active substances in the sex hormones," they pointed out.

Four years earlier evidence was presented by C. P. Rhoads in a *Bulletin of the N. Y. Academy of Medicine* (1942) to show that in rats one of the two benzene ring substances, "butter yellow," would result in the development of cancer when their diet consisted of polished rice and carrots. *If liver or yeast was added to the basal diet, no cancer occurred.* Here, clearly, was an experiment in which a constituent, rich in its contents of the vitamins of the B complex, was protective against induced cancer.

Thiamin (B₁) Deficiency

One might expect to find a vitamin deficiency in a patient who as the result of a serious illness, is in a state of malnutrition. But one of the young women examined by Ayre and Bauld, who showed evidence of malignancy in cytology smears, revealed excellent nutrition externally. She admitted, however, that she dieted constantly to keep her weight down, and analysis of her diet revealed an inadequate thiamin (B₁) intake.

"A study of thiamin physiology and metabolism reveals evidence to indicate that this substance would appear to be particularly vulnerable to intermittent or chronic depletion without gross deficiency in the diet as a whole," say Ayre and Bauld. "This tendency

[240]

would appear to depend upon the fact that little thiamin is stored in the organism and the amount is sufficient only to maintain proper life for a few days. A daily intake of thiamin is necessary and the organism absorbs only enough for the immediate needs, the excess being destroyed or excreted. More is required when alcohol is imbibed or when a high *carbohydrate* diet is taken."

". . . it is often stated," writes Dean Burk of the National Cancer Institute, "that in man alone there are well over 100 well-known and quite different kinds of cancer, usually with the implication that therefore we will have to find one or several hundred different bases for prevention and treatment, and usually without any realization that this need not necessarily be the case now that we know that all cancers studied have a characteristic metabolism in common, *a prime cause— impaired respiration of the cell.*

"And, of tremendous importance is the fact that the list of active respiratory groups includes some quite ordinary substances such as B vitamins involved in respiration (nicotinamide, riboflavin, thiamin, pantothenic acid, cobalamine) and iron salts, and some less ordinary compounds such as cytohemin and delta-amino-levulinic acid (precursor of oxygen-transferring hemins).

Value of Diet Demonstrated

Burk goes on to point out that "The precancerous lesion of the Plummer-Vinson syndrome, formerly widely prevalent in Scandinavia, has become relatively rare

[241]

there since the use, beginning in the late thirties, of some of these vitamins and iron, *added to the diet,* as a cancer preventative."

Is it possible that the answer to preventing cancer of the uterine cervix lies in increasing our intake of thiamin and other B vitamins? Here we have a clue that sheds some light on why we tend to be thiamin deficient. A recent survey by the Department of Agriculture reveals that, as a nation, we are spending much more on sweets and starches and less on fruits and vegetables.

And yet, "unless we match the excessive intake of calories with an increase in vitamins and minerals," M. I. T. nutritionist Juan M. Navia told an American Chemical Society Symposium in September, 1967, "the increased consumption of sugar and sugar products threatens our nutritional balance. Sugar," Mr. Navia said, "has been refined to such a degree that it contributes only calories to the diet, and is devoid of the vitamins and minerals essential for its metabolism." Not only sugar, but all carbohydrates, take a bite out of your body's thiamin reserves that are already dangerously overdrawn, with little coming in from your meals or snacks if you are running with the crowd.

Nature has so arranged it that, in their natural states, both cereals and sugars, and also protein foods have more than enough of the B vitamins needed for assimilation of all the carbohydrate present. But the B vitamins are removed from processed and refined grains, they are lost in high heat and they go into the vegetable cooking water which is usually discarded. So,

[242]

where can one get the thiamin that, according to Dr. H. E. Sauberlich's report published in June, 1967 in the *American Journal of Clinical Nutrition,* serves as the coenzyme in over 24 enzyme systems? Certainly not from the so-called balanced diet which so many doctors tell us will supply all of our nutritional requirements.

Brewer's Yeast, Desiccated Liver

How then can we get enough thiamin and other B vitamin factors to protect us from the terrible inroads made by cervical cancer? From brewer's yeast and desiccated liver. Ayre and Bauld tell us that the findings of various investigators using laboratory animals would appear to indicate that liver damage may be induced by dietary deficiency which reults in interference with estrogen inactivation. It was demonstrated that in female rats the liver loses its ability to inactivate estrogen in vitamin B-complex deficiency. *Addition of brewer's yeast and in one experiment desiccated liver to the diet was found to restore the inactivating mechanism.* In fact, the amount of estrogen inactivated by the liver could be controlled at will by withholding the vitamin B complex or by restoring it to the diet.

Professor Warburg proposes large scale experiments directly on humans, since the vitamins involved contain no danger. Especially after surgical operations or radiation dosage, he says, where there is much danger from metastatic growths, these vitamins should be employed, always taking pains to use very large dosages, since with B vitamins overdosage is scarcely a real problem but under-dosage could be critically unsatisfactory.

[243]

Burk says, "Such experimentation carried out on humans with relative ease and without notable risk would involve relatively little expense. It is idle to say that such experimentation, with its disarming simplicity, has really been well tried out before, because it has *not*. The more scientists who participate in such studies, the sooner will we know what can be achieved; such studies are already well under way in Germany where every physician and medical institute has received copies, written in German, of Professor Warburg's Lindau lecture of 1966 with a broad-outline description of his proposals."

Dean Burk, who made the English language translation of Dr. Warburg's study, told the Department of Pathology of New York University Medical School on November 9, 1967 that "millions of experiments in man have shown, through the effectiveness of some vitamins, that normal cell respiration is impaired if the active groups of the respiratory enzymes are insufficiently present in the food, and that cell respiration is usually repaired promptly when these groups are added to the food, or where necessary (as with cobalamine B_{12}) injected."

The first report we cited showed the relationship between estrogens which, when they are not acted upon by the liver, tend to deprive the cells of oxygen when the oxidative element thiamin is not present. It was published over 20 years ago. Its implications were apparently overlooked by the medical profession as a whole. Do you know of any physician who, when he prescribes hormones either for birth control or meno-

[244]

pause, also prescribes B vitamins? Some doctors, when they inject hormones, also inject B vitamins. Their numbers are very few.

Vitamin B Deficiency May Precede Cancer

Many people have troubles with their mouths, tongue, lips, gums. They have burning sensations, they have ulcers, boils or patches of inflammation on their gums; white spots may have appeared on the gums or insides of cheeks, their tongues are smooth and shiny or swollen and deeply fissured, the corners of their mouths have cracks or sores.

Experts have found that many such symptoms are what they term "precancerous." This does not mean that cancer is caused by these disorders. It means simply that often the bodily condition that produces such disorders in the mouth may later produce cancer. It was thought for a long time that such conditions were caused by irritation of some kind. And it is believed that cancer is often the result of irritation superimposed on just the right combination of ill-health factors to make the body susceptible to cancer.

We can report some conclusive work which seems to show that a deficiency in vitamin B is responsible for most such mouth disorders. Readers who suffer from them can take heart, for not only is there a good possibility that plenty of vitamin B will bring back good health, but the fear of cancer can be disposed of. Such mouth conditions need not be "precancerous" if you get plenty of vitamin B.

"In most cases of intra-oral cancer, there are in addi-

[245]

tion to the primary lesions, definite degenerative changes in the oral mucous membranes which obviously have antedated the malignant growth. It has long been noted that such degenerative tissue changes are found in a majority of patients with mouth cancer, and, therefore, they are commonly referred to as precancerous," say Hayes Martin, M.D., and Everett Koop, M.D., in an article in the *American Journal of Surgery* for August, 1942. Here are the medical names for some of the changes they are talking about: leukoplakia, subacute or chronic inflammation, vascular injection, atrophy or hypertrophy of the papillae, erosion of the epithelium. Most of them can be produced by chronic forms of irritation—from tobacco, venereal disease, badly fitting dentures and so forth.

It is well known, these authors say, that the B vitamins are important for mouth health. In studying 300 patients at Memorial Hospital, New York, they found that those who were suffering from mouth disorders, ranging all the way from the slightest irritation to fullblown advanced cancer of the mouth, were short on vitamin B. They found, too, that, in general, other symptoms of vitamin B deficiency accompanied the mouth symptoms in these patients. Depression and malnutrition went hand-in-hand with constipation and other digestive disorders. Interestingly enough, Drs. Martin and Koop mention fragility of finger-nails as one of the most easily recognized symptoms of vitamin B deficiency. A tendency for nails to break easily, and ridges that extend lengthwise or horizontally are further indications of lack of vitamin B.

[246]

Some Actual Conditions

Here are some of the actual mouth conditions that prevailed: *glossodynia* (a burning sensation of the tongue), chronic inflammation of the mucous membrane lining of the mouth, ulceration of the tongue, cheeks or gums, atrophy and hypertrophy of the papillae of the tongue (this means a decrease or increase in the size of the little knobs on the surface of the tongue, so that the tongue may be partly or wholly bald), fissure folding (this is a condition in which the tongue has become too large and is compressed into folds which look like crevices or fissures in its surface), *leukoplakia* (consists of white spots on the inside of the mouth. Incidentally, our authors tell us that about 50% of all men and about 10% of all women over the age of 45 have some degree of leukoplakia), *gingivitis* (bleeding from the gums), salivary changes (the mouth becomes dry and the scanty saliva becomes sticky and thick), Plummer-Vinson Disease (inflammation of the esophagus, anemia, inflammation of the tongue).

Since these are the visible changes in the lining of the mouth, our authors state that undoubtedly, farther along in the digestive tract where we cannot see them, similar disorders are prevalent. "The evidence is plain," they state, "for at least a tentative diagnosis of lack of vitamin B when an inflammatory oral mucosal lesion is associated with one or more of the following symptoms: malnutrition, mental depression, dermatoses (skin trouble), nervousness, insomnia, constipation and irregularities of the fingernails."

[247]

Which of Us Is Deficient in Vitamin B?

What is a vitamin B deficiency? Can you pick one person out of a crowd and say that he is deficient in vitamin B and pick out another and say that he is not? According to our authors, "It would be impossible to separate a group of individuals into two definite classes, one with conclusive evidences of vitamin B deficiency and the other with no evidences whatsoever. No laboratory test has been devised which furnishes an accurate basis for this determination. For this reason, there is as yet no method of determining the absolute incidence of lack of vitamin B in mouth cancer or precancer. The proof of such dietary inadequacy is found in the fact that a large percentage of patients with mouth cancer do manifest one or more of the general and local abnormalities. And that these are almost always improved by administration of vitamin B."

Then, too, there is the complicating factor that people who start out with some mouth disorder generally end up with rather serious vitamin deficiencies as well as other forms of malnutrition for the simple reason that it is so hard for them to eat. In spite of any encouragement, they avoid most carefully those foods which would contribute most to curing their deficiency—fresh raw foods—fruits and vegetables.

Drs. Martin and Koop took careful dietary surveys of hundreds of patients while they were collecting material for this article. It is, of course, difficult to find out exactly what people eat unless they are under constant and very close supervision. But the several case histories they give in the article show extremely bad

[248]

dietary habits. For instance, there was one woman who lived almost completely on gin. And, although she eventually died of "alcoholism" they say they are quite sure that her main difficulty was a lack of Vitamin B and she could have been saved, had she been given massive doses of the B vitamins.

Wide Survey Made By Physicians

Giving brewer's yeast as the best source of the B vitamins was done uniformly throughout the experimental period. And we mean large doses of brewer's yeast. The average dose was 3 tablespoons a day. In one case a man who was being treated for cancer of the tongue was given liver and yeast. Within two months he had gained a badly needed 25 pounds in weight. About a year and a half after treatment was begun he appeared to be losing ground even though he continued to take the yeast and to eat large quantities of vitamin B-rich food. So the daily intake of yeast was increased to 8 tablespoons daily "a dose which few patients can tolerate without marked nausea and diarrhea." There was tremendous improvement in his condition almost at once. From then on, so long as he maintained this enormous daily intake of yeast he remained healthy and the condition of his mouth remained good.

"These cases in which massive doses of vitamin B must be taken in order to maintain health can be explained on the basis of marked individual variations in ability, either to absorb or utilize ingested vitamins," say the authors. Among patients they studied whose

[249]

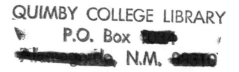

diets contained apparently enough B vitamins to keep them in fairly good health, there were some who were definitely suffering from deficiency. Although their intake of B vitamins was not far below normal, their requirement was abnormally high. It is well to remember in this connection the theories of Dr. Roger Williams of the University of Texas, who believes that alcoholism is a disease of persons who require far more vitamin B than the average person and just don't get it, no matter how good a diet they eat.

"Fad" Diets Actually Worsened Conditions

How did people fall into the practice of eating the diets that were notoriously bad? According to Drs. Martin and Koop some of these diets were prescribed by doctors for such diverse conditions as ulcer, gall bladder disease, obesity, colitis, and so forth. Some patients had blindly followed completely inadequate diets for many years firmly believing that some disorder of theirs could be cured by "dieting." Instead, they had brought on a worse condition than the one they had started out to cure. In some cases, a deficient diet brought about such loss of appetite and interest in food that the patient progressively restricted his diet still further to "those substances most easily and cheaply obtained, mainly pure carbohydrates." For instance, there was a wealthy eccentric who ate only breakfast and then took beer and onions whenever he got hungry during the rest of the day. A woman voluntarily went on an "ulcer diet" along with her husband who actually had an ulcer. A beer salesman drank beer when hungry. A traveling salesman ate only sandwiches because he was afraid of dirty food in restaurants. A woman avoided pork, fruit and eggs because certain members of her family were allergic to these foods. And so forth.

Dietary Prejudices Can Harm Health

The most frequent underlying cause of an inadequate vitamin intake lies in personality factors such as peculiar dietary prejudices based on family customs. Often deficient diets are encountered because of fear of overweight. "In most city dwellers," say our authors, "there is a tendency to eat at 'quick lunches' and drugstore counters, where green vegetables and fresh meats are replaced by carbohydrates in the form of sandwiches, ice cream, malted milk and pastry."

According to these researchers, there is little storage of excess vitamin B in the body and deficiency symptoms occur *within a few days* after withdrawal of the vitamin source. For this reason, correcting such a deficiency must be done on a daily basis. "We have found it advisable," they go on, "when using natural concentrates such as yeast and liver, to provide from five to 10 times the normal minimum requirement of thiamin and riboflavin or 30 to 45 grams (two to three tablespoons) daily of granular yeast. In exceptional cases the maximum relief cannot be obtained unless inordinately high therapeutic doses are consumed as for instance, one of our patients who ingests about 240 grams (two teacups) of brewer's yeast a day and who insists

[251]

that unless this amount is taken, marked asthenia and mental depression occur."

It is noteworthy that these doctors do not give synthetic vitamins for treatment of vitamin B deficiency. They say, "In some instances the administration of a single fraction of the vitamin B complex (thiamin, riboflavin, niacin, etc.) may cause marked improvement, but combinations of the known fractions almost always give better results." Discussing the kind of yeast to take, they deplore the use of brewer's yeast *tablets* for, they say, it is almost impossible to get enough brewer's yeast for a good big dose when you take tablets. It would require about 70 ten-grain tablets to make up the equivalent of three tablespoons of yeast.

Vitamin Intake Must Be Increased and Maintained

"It would be easier to impress both physicians and the laity," say our authors, "if it could be maintained that there is no sole cause for cancer and precancer, and that there is one simple remedy which, taken in pill form, so many times a day for a few weeks, would effect a lasting cure and a preventive of the basic abnormality. *In order to relieve avitaminosis (deficiency in B), however, the mode of life must be permanently modified, that is, the intake of vitamins must be increased and maintained as long as the patient lives.* Such a permanent regime will, in many cases, become tedious since it is not supported by the emotional stimulus which accompanies a shorter, more intense course of therapy."

The italics are ours. We put them there because this

[252]

seems to us to be the key sentence for readers in all this discussion. There is no quick and easy way to good health. There is no pill you can take to relieve any physical condition or any vitamin deficiency. Being healthy is a way of life. And if you have allowed yourself to fall into a state of diet deficiency—and most of us have—you must make a permanent change in your way of life—nothing less than this will accomplish what you want. Vitamins are something you need every day and, if you would cure a deficiency, you must decide to take vitamin supplements permanently.

Drs. Martin and Koop tell us in their summary that degenerative changes are found in the lining of the mouth in most cases of mouth cancer. The most frequent reason for these changes is a deficiency in vitamin B. Most patients are already suffering from a marked deficiency when they get to their doctor. This is aggravated by the necessarily restricted diet during the painful stage of any mouth disorder. Supplementary vitamin therapy is one successful treatment of mouth cancer or conditions that are called "precancerous." There is much evidence suggesting that the mouth symptoms are repeated farther down in the digestive tract, so it seems logical that what we say here about mouth cancer applies equally to stomach and intestinal cancer as well.

In Conclusion: Remember We Need B Vitamins

Finally, we believe readers will gather, from what we have said above, a slightly different idea about how to go about taking their B vitamins. Most of us may

[253]

need extremely large amounts of them to stay in good health. The evidence above illustrates well the reasons for taking brewer's yeast or some other purely natural food supplement rather than synthetic vitamins. Since Drs. Martin and Koop wrote their article, several more B vitamins have been discovered. They could not have been put into synthetic vitamin preparations at the time this article appeared, for their existence was unknown. But they were already in the brewer's yeast and the liver preparations and these patients benefited from them, even though they had not been discovered.

Don't be afraid to take large quantities of brewer's yeast and other completely natural food supplements rich in B vitamins, like desiccated liver and wheat germ, especially if you have distressing symptoms in mouth or digestive tract. And eat a diet high in B vitamins, too. Meat, fish, eggs, wheat germ and fresh vegetables and fruits are the best sources.

CHAPTER XXIV

Minerals May Act As Cancer Inhibitors

Why does cancer strike at one person and leave the next untouched? Why can one man's tissues reject and destroy malignant cells, while his neighbor is helpless before them? Why does cancer show a geographical distribution, with extremely low rates in some regions, like Egypt, and perhaps 20 or 30 times as much incidence in the United States?

Nobody knows the answers to these questions. But studies now being conducted in England give promise of furnishing some answers that may ultimately throw a dazzling spotlight into these murky areas of ignorance. What they have tended to show so far is that the ability to resist cancer is intimately connected with the calcium metabolism.

[255]

Calcium

Preliminary findings were published by Dr. A. Elkeles in the *British Journal of Cancer* (1963, 17, 572). They represented a clinical investigation of an idea that Dr. Elkeles first expressed in *Lancet* in 1962: that patients who had calcified atherosclerosis seemed to be singularly free from cancer. This was not 100 per cent true however, and with a fine scientific impartiality, Dr. Elkeles set out in that year to see if he could disprove his own hypothesis that calcium is related to cancer resistance. He made an intensive study of 24 patients who did have cancer, even though they showed calcification of the arteries. These, if any, could certainly eliminate the possibility of any relationship.

But the relationship was not eliminated. Instead, what Dr. Elkeles found was that even though these patients had cancers of various types, they still had demonstrably greater resistance, in that after conventional surgery they were able to survive—all 24 of them —from 5½ to 15 years. Some of them are still alive and there is no telling how long they will actually survive. But by the definition that has been accepted by the medical profession, it can be said that every single one of the 24 was "cured", since the medical criterion for a cure is survival of five years after diagnosis of cancer.

Just what the relationship may be between a high degree of calcification and cancer resistance is a question that Dr. Elkeles has not yet attempted to answer. Commenting on his work, a *Lancet* editorial (June 9,

1964) stated "Evidence is accumulating that calcium may indeed be relevant to the growth of malignant tissue. Calcium has been shown to be absent from cancer tissue (or present in only small amounts); fulminating growths are characteristically unable to take up calcium from the blood; and lack of calcium at the cell surface is responsible for the reduced adhesiveness and, perhaps, for some of the disorganized behavior of malignant cells. Thus, there are indications that, one way and another, calcium and cancer do not agree. But Elkeles has not yet established any more precise relation."

The editor of *Lancet* is perfectly right of course. Dr. Elkeles has not proved his case, nor does he claim that he has. All that he has published so far is a preliminary report which demonstrates that he could not destroy his hypothesis with evidence drawn from the tiny minority of cancer patients who also have an excess of calcium in their systems.

He would also seem to have demonstrated that, while calcium can in no way be considered a cure for cancer, it does give a powerful boost to the curative process as well as to a person's ability to resist the dread killer.

Bone Meal

It will be noted of course that Dr. Elkeles' study is dealing with the element calcium. The mineral is found in leafy vegetables, in hard water and in dairy products in good supply. But of all the foods that contain calcium, it is bone meal alone that contains it in combina-

[257]

tion with all the other trace elements in precisely the proportions in which the mammalian metabolism requires them. This makes bone meal the most assimilable form of calcium, far more of it, gram for gram, actually being absorbed into the system and utilized from bone meal than from any other source. Dr. Elkeles also makes a strong point of the ability of the tissues to absorb calcium—what he calls an affinity—playing an important role in cancer resistance. This ability is very often a question of what other trace minerals are combined with the calcium. Many mineral combinations, as they occur in bone meal, are far more absorbable to our digestive systems than the same minerals in purified form.

A fascinating explanation of what may be the relationship between the high mineral foods, and ability to resist cancer is found in the book *Chemistry of Chelation in Cancer* (Charles C. Thomas, Springfield, Illinois, 1963) by Dr. Arthur Furst, director of the Institute of Chemical Biology of the University of San Francisco. Basing his concept on a vast store of existing knowledge, Dr. Furst speculates that the way cancer develops is intimately bound up with the ability of the individual cell to produce nucleic acids that carry necessary genetic information about when and how the cell is to reproduce, the form it is to take, the limitations on its size and reproduction, and the kind of work it is to perform. That the nucleic acids control the cell in this way is rather firmly established by now. And it thus seems obvious that when cells suddenly enter into wild growth and changes in structure and function,

[258]

something has gone wrong with the nucleic acids the cell is or should be producing.

Magnesium

Dr. Furst points out that a very important role in the formation of nucleic acids is played by the trace mineral magnesium. In incredibly small amounts, this mineral (which occurs in bone meal in the proportion of 1½ milligrams to a gram) is an integral part of the nucleic acid structure. And when there is a deficiency of magnesium, he speculates, it is possible that this provides the room for a carcinogenic agent to link into the forming nucleic acid, changing its nature and as a necessary consequence, changing the nature of the cell.

"By themselves," Dr. Furst points out, "metals are unable to get into the cells; they may be transported, however, as part of a chelate system." A chelate system is a compound of two or more metals that tend to lock together because of a special affinity. Because this process alters the electrical charge, it is frequently true that a chelated compound passes more easily through intestinal walls, cell walls etc., than either of the elements of the compound can do individually. This is very definitely true of magnesium and calcium. Together, both are far more readily absorbed than either one can be separately. Although magnesium seems the more important of the two, calcium is also intimately involved in the proper formation of nucleic acids, and moreover, the magnesium does not get into the cell as it should except as part of a chelated compound with calcium.

[259]

Being thoroughly conversant with the means whereby deficiency of the important minerals calcium and magnesium can permit other, harmful minerals to leap into the cell and into the very nucleic acid pattern, Dr. Furst makes in his book a stirring plea for thorough studies of the relationship between cancer incidence and the mineral content of the soil. "In some parts of Europe a relationship was found between the number of inhabitants who developed stomach cancer and the distribution of minerals in the local soil. In some French areas a lack of magnesium oxide content seems to be reflected in a greater occurrence of cancer. Higher silicon dioxide content of the soil in some parts of the Netherlands regions seems also to be associated with a greater number of cancer patients; the effects of the high silicon concentration seems to be overcome by a high calcium oxide content. Results found may be related to the fact that tumors have a low calcium content, which may decrease the adhesiveness of these special cells and thus contribute to their increased invasiveness.

"Similar studies undertaken in Great Britain on the relationship between cancer incidence and types and percentages of trace elements in the soil have shown that chalk and limestone (high calcium) areas have low cancer rates."

Embryos Protected

Indirectly, further support for this concept can be found in the *Canadian Medical Association Journal* for May 23, 1964, in which a lengthy letter from J. H.

[260]

Davidson, M. D., points out there is some substance in the placenta that prevents cancer from being communicated to a fetus, even when the mother is suffering from an advanced stage of the disease. What can this mysterious substance be? A very thorough review article on "The Parathyroid Glands and Calcium Metabolism" by Dr. Alexander Kenny in the *World Review of Nutrition and Dietetics* (Vol. 2, 1960, Hafner Publishing Company, New York) states that the human placenta is invariably well supplied with calcium, regardless of the state of the mother's nutrition. Where the mother does not eat enough calcium, parathyroid hormone will dissolve portions of her bones in order to keep enough calcium in the placenta.

Couple this fact with the other observable fact that, even though cancer can generally spread via the blood stream, the embryo being nourished by its mother's cancer-contaminated blood will *not* contract cancer and we have another very important yardstick by which to measure just how big a role calcium may play in cancer prevention.

It should be emphasized here, as we have previously stated, that there is no reason to suppose calcium is anything like a cure for cancer. Its importance, and that of magnesium, are as natural defenses of the healthy body against the invasion of cancer-causing agents. Any one who has actually contracted cancer should certainly be under medical supervision. But perhaps the doctor involved had not yet heard of the particular areas of cancer research we have gone into in this article. Perhaps he is not aware that a high

[261]

blood serum level of the minerals provided by bone meal and other high-calcium foods might make an extremely valuable adjunct to the therapy he is using, in promoting the natural resistance of the body. In that case, it is certainly in order to call this article to his attention. And for all of us, it is an obvious precaution against the disease that is the nearest thing we have in modern times to a plague, to take steps to make up in our diets for any possible mineral deficiencies in the soil in which our plants were grown.

CHAPTER XXV

The Role of Magnesium

J. I. Rodale

Back in 1939 we first discovered the researches of Professor P. Schrumpf-Pierron, whose work is written up in the *Bulletin de l' Institut D'Egypte,* Vol. XIV, Feb. 15, 1932, and others. He talks about the *rarity of cancer in Egypt* where malignant cases are only about *one tenth that of Europe.* What is the cause? After exhaustive studies and research the Professor came to the conclusion that it was due to too much potassium and too little magnesium in the foods of Europeans. On the other hand in the *soils of Egypt* the conditions are reversed, that is, *more magnesium in relation to the potassium.*

There seems to be a definite relationship between magnesium and potash wherever it is found, whether in the soils, rocks or other places. Where there is an oversupply of potash there is always an undersupply of magnesium and vice versa. Schrumpf-Pierron studied

[263]

the cancer statistics for France in relation to the rock structure underlying its soils. It worked most uncannily. *Wherever he found an excess of potash there he discovered less magnesium and more human cancer cases.* Wherever he observed a minimum of potash he found a maximum of magnesium and less cancer cases. This means that people who eat food raised in certain soils that obtain their nutriments from the rocks which underlie them, get certain elements into their foods because of this. Such a condition would apply more to France than to the United States because in a country like France there would be more of a tendency to consume food near the point at which it is raised. But in the United States with our more advanced industrial condition where even the poorer peoples will eat winter vegetables raised in California, Florida, and elsewhere, and a great deal of citrus foods, etc. and meats that are shipped long distances, local deficiencies and unbalancings of nutritional elements may tend to be corrected to a certain extent.

"When Schrumpf-Pierron found that an excess of potassium in the rocks of a region tied in with an excess of cancer cases in that section, we should note that excess potassium means excess carbohydrates in plants grown there and therefore, reduced protein in the foods. *Farmers* should know that it is best, therefore, to use *dolomitic limestone* when they apply lime, because it *is rich in magnesium* and acts as a safety factor in relation to the potash in the soil."

Under date of May 19, 1931, Dr. Schrumpf-Pierron presented a paper, entitled "On The Cause of The

[264]

Rarity of Cancer in Egypt," which was printed in the *Bulletin of The Academy of Medicine,* and the *Bulletin of The French Assoc. For The Study of Cancer* in July 1931. The following is a digested and simplified version of it:

During the year 1931, I presented to the Academy of Medicine in Paris several papers on the rarity of cancer in Egypt, which came to the following conclusions:

1. *Cancer for Egypt is about one-tenth that of Europe and America.*

2. *In Egypt, cancer is less frequent in country fellahins than in the Egyptians who live in the towns and who have adopted Europeanized dietary habits.*

3. *The degree of malignity of Egyptian cancers is less than that of European cancers. They develop less quickly and have less of a tendency to invade neighboring tissues.*

4. *The type of cancer which is the most frequent in all the countries rich in cancer is cancer of the digestive tract, which represents 40 to 50 per cent of all cancers. In the case of Egyptians, this type of cancer is remarkably rare; in the country fellahins, practically nonexistent.*

My predecessors at l'Ecole de Medicine, Fergusson, Madden, Day, Dolbey as well as the eminent English cancer specialist, Roger Williams, have arrived at the same conclusions. Engel Bey wrote in 1908: "From these data it appears that the reputation of Egypt for comparative immunity from cancer is well founded."

What are the causes of the rarity of cancer in Egypt?

[265]

After having eliminated racial and climatic factors for reasons which can be found in my preceding papers, I said to myself that it must be looked for in an element contained in the food. It is this which led me to do research on the food of the fellahin, and I found that which characterizes the diet of the fellahin is its richness in salts of magnesium. The fellahin consumes by his food, by the water he drinks, and by the crude salt which he uses, from 2.5 to 3 grams of magnesium per day, against 4 to 5 grams of potash.

What is, by comparison, the mineralization of the average diet of the inhabitant of the towns of Europe and America? Let us look at the following:

Bread—For the populace, bread furnishes 40% of the caloric total, in the well-to-do classes only 20%. And it is always a question of bread which is relatively rich in potash, poor in minerals in general. Thus the principal contribution of magnesium is lacking.

Meat—The amount of minerals in meat is practically negligible.

Potatoes—The "industrial" varieties of potatoes at a large yield and at voluminous tubercles all show an excessive wealth of potash and are poor in magnesium. Thus, the consumption of large quantities of potatoes, such as, for example, is the case in Germany, represents an important contribution in potash.

Doughs, macaronis, etc. have the same composition as the flours from which they have been made. (Thus .5% of ashes at the maximum). Husked and polished rice is also poor in mineral elements.

Vegetables—Spinach, carrots, beets, celery, cabbage,

[266]

peas, all are rich in potash (.5%). Except for spinach, they are poor in magnesium, but contain at times as much calcium as potash. Salads have as an average .38% of potash, .08% of calcium, and .04% of magnesium.

But according to the analyses of M. Villain, the greater part of vegetables today are, compared to those of Wolff's time (1870), too poor in magnesium and relatively too rich in potash.

Fruits—Only the skins and rinds of fruits contain minerals and in particular magnesium.

Dairy Products—Milk is relatively rich in potash (.17%), in calcium (16%), poor in magnesium (.02%).

It can be thus seen that especially the whole cereals, and among these principally corn, are the ones in which there is enough magnesium. It is due to the processing and refining of foods that the world is being robbed of magnesium. Whereas the Egyptian fellahin's ratio is 2.5 to 3 grams of magnesium against 4 to 5 grams of potash a day, in Europe and America it is only ½ gram of magnesium against 2 to 4 grams of potash per day.

An intoxication of potash—an excess of potash poisons, can "kill" the soil where the food is grown. It poisons the plants, then man. Besides, several other authorities have already accused potash of producing cancer. Theis and Benedikt as well as Menetrier, have already stated that the higher amount of potash in cancerous tissue, which is a radioactive body, would activate the multiplication of cancerous cells.

P. Rosenstein and H. Kohler (from Berlin) who

[267]

have just published the results of their researches on the causes of cancer, come to the same conclusions: "If our opinion is correct, that is to say that potassium plays a preponderant role in the genesis of cancer, we will be better able to understand why the number of cancer cases has increased to such a degree; because *the generalization of the use of modern chemical fertilizers today brings to the organism of men and animals much more potash than was formerly true."*

Absence of Magnesium—It is this which permits potash to become toxic and cancerogenic. Potash is useful and indispensable to the plant as to man, but only in the case that it is associated in a favorable ratio to magnesium and calcium. Magnesium acts as a "brake for cancer" (Delbet), as much as an antitoxic of potash. This is why "the predisposition to cancer accompanies the deficit of magnesium reserves" (Dubar and Voisenet). The older the individual is, the easier the intoxication by potash, because the organism grows older and becomes poorer in magnesium than the younger organism; because this loss in magnesium decreases vitality, resistance, the power of regeneration of cells (Delbet) "provoking a sort of cellular anarchy which favors the evolution of cancerous processes" (L. Randoin). Thus one must conceive the role of magnesium as twofold: first as an antitoxin for potash and also as an antisenility element.

But why, it will be objected, are there in Europe agricultural districts where the inhabitants eat principally products of their own land, many vegetables, little meat, brown bread, etc., and where, however, we

[268]

find regular nests of cancer; villages where the cancer mortality reaches enormous proportions? Because it is a question of districts where the earth has become so poor in magnesium, or where an unreasonable chemical fertilizing made it so rich in potash, that the ratio of magnesium, potash, calcium has become unfavorable to such a point, that it leads particularly quickly to cancer. It is a question then in some way of a sur-mineralization by minerals the balance of which is unfavorable. It is thus that often one can explain the failure, and at times the clearly harmful effect, of the classic milk-vegetarian diet, which so many practitioners have been using again these past years. The magnesium content is too low.

The practical conclusions which result from our thesis are the following:

To prevent cancer and progressively diminish its frequency, two conditions should be fulfilled:

1. Agriculture should tend to produce new healthy plants, with "normal" mineralization; which can be obtained, as proved by M. Villain, by a regeneration of the earth with the aid of appropriate fertilizers, under a systematic control of the mineralization of cultivated vegetables. It is a question of a new science, which must be inspired with the fundamental principle *that abnormal mineralization of an alimentary plant logically has its repercussion on the mineral balance of animals and men who feed themselves on it;* that besides, the more the mineralization is "normal," the more the alimentary quality, if not the yield of the plant is

[269]

raised; that finally, in agriculture, quality must never be sacrificed to quantity.

2. Modern alimentary hygiene must greatly modify its principles and above all detach itself from the too narrow concept of "caloric worth" of an aliment as the only measure of its "nutritive worth." The overly civilized world feeds itself poorly. Without being obliged to return to the quasi-animal diet of the fellahin, it should relearn to mineralize itself normally. Thus, it is above all a *bread reform* which should be imposed, that is, certain varieties of wheat grown that are richer in magnesium than others. But the safest cereal is corn (maize) in which the proportion of magnesium is quite high. Corn is the magnesium aliment *par excellence.*

Even when it grows on less favorable soil, less rich in magnesium than Egyptian soil, corn still always contains a relatively large amount of magnesium, little potash and calcium, and a lot of phosphoric acid.

In the southern countries, where corn is the base of the diet of the people, cancer is relatively rare. It is very rare where the corn is consumed integrally, as is done by the fellahin in Egypt. If colored people in the United States show less cases of cancer than whites, it is not because the dark race is refractory, as has been said, but very probably because the American negroes have retained the African habit of eating corn.

One can state that the problem of cancer and many other illnesses depends mainly on the bread in the diet. There must be a reorganization of agricultural methods, especially with regard to the kind of fertilizers used, and a change of concept in the food factories and

[270]

bakeries. It is urgent that we act because cancer is terribly on the increase.

With regard to fertilizers, the organic method, using no chemical fertilizer, but composts made from animal manures and vegetable matter, insures against the over-application of potash to the soil. Dolomite limestone, rich in magnesium, should be used.

This article is another proof that opposition to the eating of bread is sound. *We are for corn all the way.* Biscuits of it can be made without the addition of wheat flour. Also, corn mush can be delicious. Corn pancakes can be made with corn meal, eggs, wheat germ flakes and black-strap molasses. I have tried them. They are delicious. For children, some bone meal powder can be mixed in. Bone meal also is extremely rich in magnesium.

The rate of cancer in the southern U.S. is much lower than in the North. This may be due to less heating smoke in the atmosphere, and to some extent to the great use of corn in the southern diet.

Here are some figures:

In 1961 the cancer death rate per 100,000 population was 178.3 for the New England states, compared with 128.2 for the South Atlantic states. The Middle Atlantic states (New York, New Jersey, Pennsylvania) had a rate of 180.5 compared with 127.7 in the East South Central states. The highest rate for the continental U.S. was in New York (186.6) and the lowest in New Mexico (78.8).

More corroboration. In 1958, the last year for which

[271]

a figure is available, the Egyptian rate was 28.5, and the U.S. rate 146.9.

Yet in spite of the statistical confirmation of what Schrumpf-Pierron pointed out half a century ago, there didn't seem to be any modern scientists interested in following up on his work. It seemed for a long while that the magnesium question would be one more open door through which science had refused to look.

Suddenly, this year, all that changed. At the annual meeting of the Federation of American Societies for Experimental Biology, 1968, an inspiring report was made by Dr. P. Bois, M.D., Ph.D., the chairman of the department of anatomy of the University of Montreal. Dr. Bois told the FASEB that he is now searching for the connection between magnesium deficiency and cancer.

If a scientist finds a spontaneous tumor in a rat, he considers it a rarity. Somehow, ordinary rodents almost never develop cancer. Even causing tumors artificially can be a challenge to the scientist. Yet, a group of Canadian researchers headed by Dr. Bois has discovered that merely eliminating the trace mineral magnesium from the diets of rats can trigger tumor growth within an average of 64 days. The original tumors invariably develop in the thymus gland, but if the diet deficiency is not corrected, cancer will develop in other parts of the body, and eventually lymphoid leukemia will develop.

In an interview with us, Dr. Bois gave some of his theories on why magnesium deficiency leads to the tumor growth. "Magnesium is essential for numerous

[272]

enzymic processes in the cell as well as for the integrity of structure of chromosomes and nucleic acids. Withdrawing magnesium may lead to mutation of those chromosomes, and the mutation may lead to tumor growth," he said. But he also added that such chromosomal mutation has not yet been found.

Another theory is that low magnesium levels produce high calcium levels and a loss of phosphate. Perhaps it is not the magnesium itself, but one of those other changes which is directly related to tumor growth.

Dr. Bois' study is the second of its type in the medical literature. The first was performed last year (1967) in Chicago by a group that found that a diet containing as little as five milligrams of magnesium per 100 grams of food produced myogenic leukemia in animals after one year.

But, in applying his findings to human cancers, Dr. Bois is pioneering in a new area of research. An admitted nonconformist, Bois somewhat shyly acknowledges that his belief that a magnesium deficiency can cause cancer is far off the beaten track of most cancer theories. But there is no quarreling with his discovery that rats—which just don't get cancer—do develop tumors when magnesium is taken from their diets.

"There is a lot of magnesium in humans," says Bois, "in blood and bone and urine. All foods have magnesium in them. But if your diet is too high in fats or lipids, you may need more than ordinary amounts of magnesium because you lose too much of the mineral in those substances." Bois points out that magnesium is still a mystery in many ways. Its exact function and

[273]

how much is needed are still not known. It has only been in recent years that scientists have been able to measure magnesium in the blood at all. Before then, magnesium was considered a useless mineral.

Working with the Institute of Microbiology and the Cancer Institute of Notre Dame Hospital, both in Montreal, he is establishing magnesium levels of all hospital patients. When asked whether he felt that, in spite of the wide variety of dietary sources of magnesium, humans could still suffer a deficiency in that mineral, Dr. Bois said, "Yes, I certainly do." Much recent research indicates a general dietary deficiency in magnesium in the U.S. and Europe.

CHAPTER XXVI

Vitamin C and the Cancer Cell

W. J. McCormick, M.D.

That the cancer cell, per se, is not malignant is shown by the fact that even after metastasis to distant parts of the organism it continues to exercise in degree its normal genetic function. For instance, secondary breast tumors have been found to secrete milk, secondary gastric tumors to secrete hydrochloric acid and pepsin, secondary liver tumors to secrete bile, etc. In our opinion the real malignancy lies with the unwitting host in his or her violation of the basic laws of hygiene.

Our observations have led us to the conclusion that the major cause of vitamin-C deficiency in our modern civilization may be the well-nigh universal tobacco and alcohol addiction. *The smoking habit* not only militates against normal nutritional practice, but actually neutralizes or destroys to a great extent what little vitamin

C is taken in food. We have found by clinical and laboratory means that the smoking of one cigarette, as ordinarily inhaled, tends to neutralize in the body about 25 mg. of vitamin C, or the content of an average-sized orange. This reciprocal effect is due to the pronounced chemical action of ascorbic acid as a reducing agent. Our findings in this respect have been confirmed in general by independent research in the U.S.A. and in Europe. On the basis of our hypothesis these findings would explain the phenomenal increase in lung cancer in smokers in recent years.

This new theory of the causal relationship of vitamin-C deficiency in cancer suggests the possibility that all physical and chemical cancerogens may act indirectly by bringing about or exaggerating a latent deficiency of vitamin C. A comparable situation has prevailed regarding alcohol. For many years it was thought that alcohol was the specific cause of peripheral neuritis in the alcoholic subject, but it is now known that deficiency of vitamin B$_1$ is the culpable agent, the alcohol acting indirectly by increasing the body requirement of this vitamin. However, alcohol, as now being exploited along with tobacco in intensive advertising, is like adding insult to injury or compounding a felony.

Recently the Sloan-Kettering Institute reported a series of experimental transplants of live cancer cells in human subjects in an effort to get answers to the following questions: "Why will cancer strike one American in four, and why will the other three not get cancer? What are the differences between the cancer-prone and the cancer-free? Why does a tumor smoulder

[276]

in one human, grow slowly but steadily in another, flame wildly through the body of a third? Why does a cancer—very rarely, but demonstrably—stop growing, melt, disappear in some patients? Why does cancer growth, in other patients, seem at times temporarily checked, and then why does it accelerate again? Is there immunity to cancer? If so, is it something that exists in the cancer-free but is lacking—or destroyed— in the cancer victim? Are there at least partial natural defenses against cancer? Can they be identified, studied, stimulated, increased, created artificially or borrowed to protect the potential cancer victim?—or rescue those attacked?"

Cancer Transplantation

To begin with, they transplanted cancer tissue under the skin of the forearm in 15 advanced cancer cases. In every case the cancer implants "took," grew vigorously and spread, for periods ranging from six weeks to six months, before they were removed by surgery. Obviously these subjects were completely lacking in resistance to cancer. For comparison, another group of 14 willing subjects (inmates of Ohio State Penitentiary)—normally healthy and cancer-free—were given similar injections of the same stock of cancer cells, and in every case there was an overwhelming defense reaction, and within four weeks almost all the cancer tissue had been destroyed.

In these studies no cognizance was given to the nutritional background or living habits of the subjects and no correlation in this respect was envisaged. It is our belief that if such an assessment had been made a better approach to the solution of the problem would have been achieved. However, these experiments seem to confirm the concept of a systemic or metabolic etiology in cancer.

We now wish to review a study of the surgical curability of breast cancer reported by Haagensen *et al* from the laboratory of surgical pathology of the College of Physicians and Surgeons, Columbia University, New York City. Their study included the follow-up of 241 breast-cancer patients treated by surgical removal of breasts from 1935 through 1948, with a follow-up from 10 to 24 years. After excluding from this study any unusual types, there remained 204 cases designated as common types of breast cancer. These were again divided into two groups:

(A) *those with well delimited, rounded or lobulated contour,* (B) *those with serrated, grossly irregular, often stellated periphery, showing radical projections into the surrounding tissue. The well delimited group yielded 46 tumors and the grossly irregular type yielded 158 tumors. There was a correlation between these types and their curability at ten or more years—the well delimited group had a cure rate of 80% as contrasted to only 38% for the irregular tumors.*

The marked difference in curability, or so-called malignancy, of these two types of tumors, as viewed by these authors, was in no way related to the living habits of the subjects, but rather to the assumed intrinsic degree of malignancy of the component cells. On the contrary, we regard the marked difference in conformity

[278]

and curability of these two types of tumors as directly related to the nutritional status of the subjects, with special reference to vitamin-C status, and adequate maintenance of which, with resultant maintenance of normalcy of the intercellular cement substance (collagen) determining the normal stability of the involved cells, and the consequent degree of potential cancer development.

We now review a still more recent study on the "Relative Influence of Conservative and Radical Surgery on the Survival of Patients With Breast Cancer" by Devitt, J. E., of the Ottawa (Canada) Civic Hospital. Eight hundred and forty-eight patients were included in this five-year follow-up study, 444 of which were eligible for a 10-year follow-up. The operable patients were divided into a radical mastectomy, with or without pre-operative or post-operative irradiation, and the latter having had simple mastectomy, with or without excision of the adjacent lower axillary lymph glands; in nine cases there was only a simple excision of the tumor.

In these cases some of the surgeons routinely practiced radical surgery in all cases, while a few performed simple procedures routinely, simple mastectomy being usually reserved for the "poor-risk" patients and the elderly. In "summary and conclusions" this author states that "radical surgery provided no advantage in crude five and 10-year survival compared with conservative surgery," and that the latter "exerted a statistically significant advantage in patients with proved metastases and in premenopausal women."

[279]

Additional Support?

This review, we think, would give additional support to our hypothesis if a correlated study of the vitamin-C status of the subjects had been made to determine the possible relationship of associated connective-tissue status which could prevent metastasis by maintaining collagenous stability in the axillary lymph nodes, and other connective tissues throughout the organism.

It is not expected that our hypothesis, as advanced herein, will lead to a cure for cancer in its advanced stages, but the prospects for prophylaxis and curbing or containing of the disease in its early stages seem most encouraging. As an aid in the solution of this vital problem it is suggested that bio-chemical studies of the vitamin-C status should be made on all middle-aged subjects, and nutritional guidance given accordingly, in the hope of at least effecting prophylaxis of this terrible disease. "An ounce of prevention is worth a pound of cure."

Summary

We submit herewith additional evidence in support of our previously advanced hypothesis that deficiency of vitamin C, by bringing about disintegration of epithelial and connective tissue relationships, owing to liquefaction of the intercellular cement substance (collagen), results in a breakdown of orderly cellular arrangement, which could be the precursor to cancer.

The recent observations of Gillman et al. on collagen and connective tissue changes in the dermis of chronically injured areas are cited, indicating formation of

[280]

"pseudo-elastic tissue." They suggest that similar collagenous degenerative skin conditions which frequently become cancerous, and that thus degenerated dermal collagen may play an important role in cancer pathogenesis.

These authors in no way implicated vitamin C deficiency in the etiology of these degenerative changes, but we believe that such nutritional deficiency may be the primary cause of precancerous degeneration.

[281]

CHAPTER XXVII

Vitamin A Protects
Against Cancer

What may turn out to be one of the most important pieces of research in the history of modern medicine was unveiled in Tokyo in October 1966 at the Ninth International Cancer Congress. Dr. Umberto Saffiotti, a pathologist at the Chicago Medical School, reported that he had virtually 100 per cent success in giving lung cancer to laboratory animals by exactly the same means that the disease is supposed to be caused in humans. In identical animals, however, he was able to reverse the process and render the animals immune to cancer-causing chemicals he used on them, by giving them vitamin A as well.

The importance of such a discovery is a matter that it would be impossible to overestimate.

Dr. Saffiotti himself, in the manner typical of scientists, warned that his findings were not yet conclusive, and while he felt that they might "possibly lead to results of practical significance for the prevention of lung cancer," he also felt that such results had not yet been achieved.

Let us examine the technique of his laboratory study, however, and try to evaluate it for ourselves.

Top Expert

In the first place, there is little or no possibility that Dr. Saffiotti could be mistaken about whether he was truly dealing with cancer. A pathologist is a laboratory technician whose specialty is the examination of diseased tissue and the precise determination of what disease, if any, is present. A pathologist at a leading American medical school, which is what Dr. Saffiotti is, is a man whose opinion would be accepted without question anywhere in the world.

So we can assume that the Doctor knows what he is talking about when he says that he had practically 100 per cent success in giving lung cancer to hamsters. Why hamsters? Because these animals never contract lung cancer by natural means. Therefore, to stimulate the development of cancer in their lungs could not be supposed questionable and possibly the result of a normal occurrence happening simultaneously. If the hamsters got lung cancer at all, it could only be because of what Dr. Saffiotti was doing to them.

What he was doing was subjecting their lungs to benzpyrene, the hydrocarbon that is believed to be the chief cancer-causing chemical in cigarette smoke as well as in automobile exhausts, and smoke from the

[283]

coal and oil fires of home and factory. This material was permitted to fasten itself to inert particles of dust, in exactly the same way it does in the atmosphere. The dust was then placed in the windpipes of hamsters.

The particles were found to lodge in the lower portion of the lungs. Cell fluid in the lungs washed the dust particles, separating out the benzpyrene and dispersing the cancer-causing material throughout the lung tissue. When the benzpyrene reached the cells lining the bronchi—the tubular passages through which air is channeled into the lungs—the cells began to grow and divide in a rapid, irregular manner. It was soon evident that all the animals that were, in effect, subjected to the same air pollutants as a smoker and city dweller, had developed lung cancer.

Vitamin A Protects

It is well known that vitamin A is intimately connected with the health and functioning of the lining of the bronchi. Dr. Saffiotti experimented with giving large doses of vitamin A to his laboratory hamsters to see if that would have any affect on the rate or manner of development of the lung tumors.

And what an effect it had! ". . . when he also feeds them vitamin A, very few come down with lung tumors," according to the Associated Press report of his paper.

Dr. Saffiotti was careful to warn that he did not intend his report to be taken as advice for smokers to start dosing themselves with massive amounts of vitamin A. He also warned that excess vitamin A can be

[284]

harmful. Vitamin A, as is true of all the oil-soluble vitamins whose surpluses are stored in the liver rather then being excreted, cannot be taken without limit. What your personal limit is depends very much on how you react to the vitamin. We have reason to believe that up to 50,000 International Units a day are safe for any adult. According to the Merck Manual, "With one possible exception, this rare condition (hypervitaminosis A) thus far has been described only in patients receiving more than 100,000 units a day." The symptoms of an excess of vitamin A are described as sparse coarse hair, a dry rough skin and cracked lips as early signs, followed by severe headache and generalized weakness. Bones may become decalcified, the liver enlarged, and localized hemorrhages occur.

So at the first sign of coarsening falling hair and cracked dry lips or skin, if you are taking very large amounts of vitamin A, we would recommend that you reduce your intake. However, there is no reason to suppose that such reactions could occur in you if you are taking a sensible daily intake of 100,000 units or less.

In fact, we see no reason to believe that any more than that same amount should ever be necessary to promote one's resistance to cancer. As a matter of fact, it was reported at the same International Cancer Congress that in Japan the new dietary practice of drinking milk has been found to exert a protective effect against the development of stomach cancer. There is little doubt in our minds that such protection as milk exerts is because of the large vitamin A content of this otherwise unwholesome drink. Yet in the amount of milk

[285]

that an adult would normally drink in one day, there is far less than 100,000 units of vitamin A or even than 50,000. If milk—a source of vitamin A far inferior to halibut or cod liver oil—can exert a protective effect against cancer, then there is no need for anyone ever to think he requires massive doses of the vitamin for the protection it affords. A normal substantial amount such as you would take anyway simply to maintain good health should be enough to do the trick.

Still another study of the protective effect of this vitamin deals with the papilloma, a special type of abnormal growth or neoplasm that is very widespread indeed. When it appears on the skin, where it can be seen, it resembles the nipple of the female breast, which is the source of its name. These growths on the skin are usually harmless except for the annoyance they cause. But they can also occur internally, causing dangerous obstruction of delicate passages such as the digestive tract, and in many cases bleeding and inducing anemia. Internal or external, they are capable of turning malignant.

If you have one or more papillomas, it is nothing to go into a panic about. They are probably harmless. Yet they represent a danger and it is far better to get rid of them than to ignore them. It was an exciting development, therefore, when we recently found in *Cancer Research* (February, 1967) an article by Ronald E. Davies of the Skin and Cancer Hospital of Temple University in Philadelphia, indicating that vitamin A has been found in laboratory research to be an excellent treatment for getting rid of papillomas.

[286]

The study set up by Dr. Davies employed large numbers of a particular species of mouse—the rhino mouse —because the species is known to be especially susceptible to the development of papillomas on the skin. Such mice were fed a diet providing full nutrition in every respect except that it contained no vitamin A. Half of them were fed 100 International Units of vitamin A daily, while the other half continued to get none of this vitamin, as a control. All animals had a cancer-causing chemical applied to their skins.

Vitamin Preserved Youth

The first observation made by Dr. Davies was that the animals receiving the vitamin A had pinker skin with fewer wrinkles on it than did those on the diet deficient in this vitamin. They were also found to be more active and not to relapse into inactivity (old age) as soon as those not receiving the vitamin. There was, however, no frank indication of a vitamin A deficiency in the control group of mice. This confirmed earlier observations that animals (and perhaps people) receiving a good nutritional supply of all other vitamins including E, take a long time to develop any signs that are presently recognized as symptoms of deficiency disease. There is a good chance that this is actually a deficiency in the present state of medical knowledge, however, for it was also observed of these mice that in response to application of a cancer-causing chemical, those well supplied with vitamin A developed fewer papillomas, and after developing them, were able to

[287]

break down and eliminate more of those that had been developed.

It was thus demonstrated that A played a definite role in enabling these mice both to resist the formation of these tumors and also to overcome and eliminate the tumors once they had formed. So it is entirely possible that lowered resistance of the skin to tumors is one sign, not yet recognized, of deficiency in vitamin A.

It seems remarkable to us that as recently as a year ago the medical profession was sharply attacking this vitamin and trying to persuade people to take less of it. Yet within the past year there have emerged the research reported above and another, even more significant, indicating that vitamin A may well be one of our primary protections against cancer and that what we may all need is more of it, rather than less.

CHAPTER XXVIII

Blood Sugar and Cancer

If American medicine ever reaches the point of being able to greatly reduce the incidence of the major diseases, heart disease, cancer, high blood pressure and such, we have a good idea who the hero of the accomplishment is going to be. In our entire country we know of only one group of doctors, and those under the leadership of only one individual, seriously concerned with studying how candidates for illness may be discovered before they become sick and thus guided to remain healthy.

The scientific group consists of brilliant young doctors and dentists working at the University of Alabama Medical Center in Birmingham, led by Emanuel Cheraskin, M.D., D.M.D., Chairman of the Department of Oral Medicine. In truly remarkable numbers over the past years, reports have been flowing from this research group of unusual and highly significant discoveries in the realm of predictive medicine.

They are studies of a type that had to be given the

[289]

new name *predictive medicine* to distinguish them from preventive medicine which is misnamed, being concerned largely with the earlier diagnosis of disease rather than its prevention. It is the predictive group that is truly concerned with prevention as we understand it, aiming at the examination and testing of healthy people to discover those who are more likely to contract an illness in the future, so that they may be guided in ways to avoid it. The concept is a foreign one to most doctors who are concerned only with treating sickness and have no interest in the healthy. Thus it must have come as something of a bombshell to the American Medical Association when Dr. Cheraskin reported to the annual convention in June, 1966 on one small aspect of his work.

Unexpected Cancer Clue

The remarkable burden of his report was that a study of the carbohydrate metabolism—fundamentally of the way the system reacts to an overload of glucose —can give significant indications of whether or not the person being examined will develop cancer in the future.

What Professor Cheraskin and his associates did was to take advantage of the annual diabetes detection drive in Birmingham, as well as the availability of dental patients at the Department of Oral Medicine, to gather what most doctors would consider unrelated statistics and see if a correlation could be established between them. They studied two groups of dental patients, one comprising 120 and the other 170 persons, all of them well by normal medical criteria. 362 more people were examined in the course of the diabetes detection drive for 1964.

According to Dr. Cheraskin, "Several points warrant particular attention. Firstly, the higher the fasting blood glucose, the higher are the values for the rest of the tolerance pattern. Secondly, the higher the initial mean value, the less is the decline in blood glucose after 30 minutes. . . . Lastly, and most importantly, one can predict, within limits, from *small* differences at the fasting level the remainder of the glucose tolerance test patterns."

In other words, although a lengthy and cumbersome procedure, bothersome to the patient, is ordinarily used to determine the characteristics of the carbohydrate metabolism, it has been found that only the first step in this procedure is usually enough to give a clear indication of how the rest of the test is going to work out.

The figures for blood glucose were then compared with a different set of figures for the same groups, to check on the incidence of tumors. A correlation was found with age, as might have been expected, but also with the incidence of a high blood glucose level. In the oldest group, those above the age of 60, 22 per cent of those with the higher blood glucose levels had tumors as compared with only six per cent in the lower blood glucose group.

Checking back on the younger groups, the variation was not so sharp in the 30 to 59 year olds, but still existed in the ratio of two to one. Below the age of 30 there were no tumors in either group.

[291]

Early Predictiveness

"The important point to be underscored is that small variations in blood glucose provide some measure of predictiveness," stated Dr. Cheraskin. What it comes down to is a strong indication that those whose metabolisms are unable to rapidly clear the blood of an excess of sugar are distinctly more likely to develop tumors in later age than those whose blood clearing mechanism is more efficient. Furthermore, a simple determination of the fasting blood sugar level may well be enough to unveil this entire pattern.

Dr. Cheraskin presented this report to the AMA, of course, in the hope that additional groups of doctors would be inspired to check it and either corroborate or refute it. It is, after all, a fantastically hopeful possibility to think that some day a doctor may be able to take a specimen of blood from a young man in perfect health and by determining the blood sugar level, know what probability there is that this healthy young man will develop cancer in 20 or 30 years. Given such a predictive tool, there is every possibility that the doctor could help his patient to avoid ever contracting cancer, or at the very least, would check him frequently enough to be able to make early diagnosis.

It is the kind of tool many in the medical profession claim to have been searching and praying for. Has anyone followed up on the lead of Dr. Cheraskin and his associates?

We wonder.

[292]

CHAPTER XXIX

Can Cancer Be Prevented?

J. I. Rodale

First let us look at our problem. How prevalent is cancer? Here are figures showing how many persons per 100,000 population in the U. S. died of cancer from 1900 to 1959:

1900	64
1910	76
1920	83
1925	92
1930	97
1935	108
1940	120
1945	127
1947	132
1959	147

An analysis of these figures should make one question the oft-repeated statements one encounters in newspapers, magazines, books and the radio, that the mortality figures show that we are getting healthier. Every year shows a small but persistent increase over the

[293]

preceding one. It is an increasing tendency that shows no desire to let up. When I bring these figures to the attention of physicians or to some laymen the invariable answer is that these cancer statistics are misleading. They say that due to better diagnostic techniques more and more cases show up in the statistics which were formerly attributed to other diseases. Therefore it must be expected that the figures *will* show an increase and that we must not be alarmed about it. However, *that* excuse has now been worked threadbare. I have heard that argument for the last 30 years, but anyone who will investigate will find that may have been true in 1910 or even in 1920, but since then, diagnosis has made so much progress that around 1930 to 1935 it had become more or less perfect and the medical profession became proud of their brilliant achievements in this field. So for all practical purposes we reached a point, let us say, 20 or 30 years ago when diagnosis improved to such an extent that any further improvement would show up only in tiny, fractional decimal points.

Is Life Expectancy Increasing?

Another reason is given, that since more persons are attaining to a higher age, and that since cancer is a disease affecting older persons, naturally it would be expected that there would be a gradual increase in cancer deaths per hundred thousand of population. There are two parts to this assumption and both are incorrect. First, are there really more older persons? The mortality figures are only figures and sometimes

[294]

figures can be misleading. Do we really have a greater life expectancy? *Time* magazine of Dec. 4, 1944 said: "In the past 44 years, past 65 life expectancy has increased only slightly. Women (white) of 65 can now expect to live longer than they could have in 1900; male expectancy has increased only half a year." This apparent discrepancy between the actual and what the public thinks is so, has to do with babies that used to die due to poor hygiene. It is due also to other conditions that do not affect *you*. You are not a baby that died in childbirth or in the first few years of life.

Cancer Is Not Caused by Old Age

The second error is the supposition that cancer is a disease of old age. Then why did the Metropolitan Life Insurance Company say the following in a release to the press February 18, 1949? "With the virtual conquest of the common childhood diseases, cancer now ranks high among the causes of death of youngsters, according to the statisticians of the Metropolitan Life Insurance Company. In the company's experience, cancer recently had accounted for one out of every nine deaths from disease at ages 1 to 14 years, while as late as 1930 the ratio was only one out of every 50. Since that year the death rate from cancer among children insured in the Industrial Department has increased about 40 per cent." And now it is skyrocketing.

Professor Hoffman who is mentioned later on in this article said in the book there quoted: "After many years' thoughtful consideration and exhaustive statistical study, I am fully convinced that the apparent

[295]

increase in cancer is real, and not to be explained away by changes in the age or constitution, or improvement in diagnoses." Nothing will be gained by arguing. Let's tackle the problem and argue afterward. We must realize that in the civilized world today we are in the midst of a dread curse and American brains must do something about it. When we are faced with figures which show that from Pearl Harbor to V-J Day 294,-476 American soldiers and sailors were killed, but that during the same period 607,193 Americans died of cancer, we can better visualize what the cold cancer statistics mean, that it is an emergency situation, a crisis, which demands bold, aggressive treatment. A statistician studying the trend of these cancer increases must come to the conclusion that if the tendency is not curbed half the population will be killed off by cancer in the next 50 to 150 years.

Prevention or Cure?

I would like to mention the work of the late Dr. Frederick L. Hoffman who was connected with the Prudential Insurance Company of America and with the Biochemical Research Foundation of the Franklin Institute of Philadelphia. He was a medical man of high repute who traveled all over the world studying cancer to see if he could obtain a clue to its causation. He devoted his life to it. In 1915 The Prudential Press published his book of 826 pages entitled, "The Mortality from Cancer Throughout the World." In 1937 The Williams and Wilkins Company, conservative medical publishers of Baltimore, Md., published his

767 page book called "Cancer and Diet," in which he quotes much evidence and the work of many physicians who hold that diet is an important element in cancer.

Very early in the book Dr. Hoffman becomes suspicious of commercial fertilizers. I am going to quote from his work:

Artificial Chemicals and Artificial Foods

"The food supply for this population (alluding to urban communities) is therefore naturally becoming more and more artificial and modified by a wide range of processes, some of which unquestionably react injuriously on the human organism. There is another factor involved to which hardly any attention has been called and that is the nature of the food supply itself which is being altered as the result of alterations in the nature of the soil in which the food is raised. This applies particularly to the composition of the mineral constituents of the soil which to an increasing extent are being modified by the addition of artificial fertilizers which also are becoming more and more chemical and artificial in contrast to the use of natural manures in the earlier days, when the soil retained most of its original fertility and growth producing capacity. In other words, any one of the principal food products consumed at the present time does not by any means represent the same natural mineral composition of say 50 years ago. . . .

"Granting that the prevention of soil exhaustion is the function of fertilizers, their effect on human consumption has attracted little attention. Since our body

[297]

is precisely what it feeds upon, chemical alterations must have affected human development and biological activities to an extent well deserving of more thoughtful consideration. The composition of foodstuffs now raised for farm animals has many years received close attention but the chemical composition of human foodstuffs has been treated with indifference. We are still of the belief that it is immaterial from what soil or sources our foodstuff is derived although the evidence is overwhelmingly to the effect that measurable differences occur which may have a serious consequence when the process is extended over a lifetime.

"As the result of the introduction of chemical fertilizers there has been a marked increase in the crop production. The average amount of wheat in bushels per acre has increased from 9.9 in 1886 to 27.3 in 1958. The relative yield per acre varies, of course, widely for different sections of the country, having been so high as 28 bushels in Arizona and as low as 5.3 bushels in North Dakota. These figures are for 1931. It is reasonable inference that the nutritional qualities, particularly mineral content, must vary proportionately to the use of chemical fertilizers in different sections, but I am not aware of any data to substantiate this conclusion at the present time. What is true of wheat is true of other grains or vegetables that enter into the food consumption of the American people. Everywhere efforts are made to increase the yield per acre but what the effect of this hazard is on the mineral or vitamin content of the food is not revealed.

[298]

"The foregoing conclusion can also be applied to animal husbandry and dairying. It is to my mind an open question if there is not a substantial difference in milk supplied by cows artificially stimulated to a milk yield far above the average. Again the same conclusion may be applied to artificially fed steers and pigs."

All of the above shows independent, creative thinking, for it was written long before Sir Albert Howard's writings on the organic method were available to the public. Dr. Hoffman quotes from the Yearbook of Agriculture for 1932 to show that in the earlier days of the use of commercial fertilizers the fertilizer was not as concentrated and soluble as it later became, but was mixed with waste or byproducts of industry, so that equal tonnages by weight would mean more chemical potency in the commercial product of the last twenty or thirty years. He then quotes from the 1932 Yearbook:

"The American farmer, in his agricultural operations, applies 8,000,000 tons of fertilizers annually. It is frequently pointed out that this is an average application of 40 pounds for each acre of land under cultivation in this country, as contrasted with 500 pounds for The Netherlands, where intensive farming is generally followed."

Artificial Chemicals and Incidence of Cancer

Dr. Hoffman did not attempt to discuss the effect of so much commercial fertilizers on the health of the people of The Netherlands so I looked up the com-

[299]

parative cancer statistics for the United States and that country taken from Hoffman's book, "The Mortality from Cancer Throughout the World." Here are figures for 1900, 1910, and 1955:

U. S.	Holland	Italy
1900—64	91	52
1910—76	106	65
1955—146.5	159.8	128

Note the higher rates for Holland. Observe the lower cancer rate for Italy where extremely small amounts of artificial fertilizers were used.

The late Dr. Max Gerson of New York City, a cancer specialist had this to say at a hearing in Washington relating to Bill No. S.1875 held on July 1, 2 and 3, 1946, to authorize the Government to sponsor cancer research, which was not passed:

"The fundamental damage starts with the use of artificial fertilizer for vegetables and fruits as well as for fodder. Thus the chemically transformed vegetarian and meat nourishment, increasing through generations, transforms the organs and functions of the human body in the wrong direction.

"Another basic defect lies in the waste of excrements of the cities. Instead of returning the natural manure to the fruit-bearing soil, it is led into the rivers, killing underwater life. The natural cycle is interrupted and mankind has to suffer dearly for the violation. Life in forest and wilderness should teach us the lesson.

"But we can regain the lost defense and healing power if we return as close as possible to the laws of nature as they are created."

[300]

Dr. George Miley of the Gotham Hospital, New York City, who worked with Dr. Gerson on some of these cases, testified at the hearing as follows:

"We do know experimentally that diet definitely does influence cancer. There is a lot of experimental work done, very good work done to substantiate that. . . . It is reasonable to assume that the closer one's diet is to nature and the soil, with fresh fruit from the trees and fresh vegetables directly from the garden, the nearer one is to normal health."

I want to quote also the *New York Times* of December, 1940. I do not have the record of the particular day. It said:

"According to Dr. Alexander Brunschwig of the University of Chicago, in the current national bulletin of the American Society for the Control of Cancer, there is experimental evidence to suggest that in animals, at least, inadequate diets may serve as adjuvants to the action of certain cancer-producing compounds.

"An illustration of this point is the recent work of Kinosita, the Japanese pathologist, working at the Memorial Hospital, New York, who has shown that when rats are fed an adequate, well-balanced diet, the ingestion of cancer-producing substance known as 'butter yellow' is innocuous. However, when the rats are maintained upon an inadequate diet, especially lacking in vitamins, the ingestion of this chemical causes inflammatory changes in the liver followed by cancer of this organ.

"Such experiments, if they can at all apply to man" states Dr. Brunschwig, "would suggest that while an

[301]

adequate, well balanced diet does not in any way insure against the development of cancer, it does contribute to the maintenance of a general normal body economy and in this way might tend to obviate the progress of other diseases or pathologic conditions which might themselves favor the development of cancer.

"It is perhaps not too far-fetched to state that when a better understanding of the mechanism of cancer development in man is obtained, the factor of diet may assume greater importance in attempts at prophylaxis (prevention) and control of the disease than can now, in our present state of knowledge, be the case."

Is Cancer Related to Artificial Fertilizers?

When the Nazis marched into Austria they drove out one of the world's greatest cancer authorities—Dr. Ernst Freund. Dr. Freund's researches—carried on for years—are based on the theory that "cancer is caused not by infection or irritation, but by false digestive processes." Frederick Pearson, an American millionaire, once saw a friend die in agony from cancer. He was profoundly shocked by the sight, and swore he would spend his last cent if necessary to see cancer wiped out. Frederick Pearson is apparently as good as his word, for he formed a research institute in Vienna, placing Dr. Freund in charge. When the Nazis turned Dr. Freund out, Pearson had the costly equipment as well as Dr. Freund transported to London.

Take the case of the late Dr. John R. Davidson, of Winnipeg, Manitoba, who during his entire professional life specialized in cancer work. Let me quote Dyson Carter, who wrote in "Saturday Night," a newspaper published in Toronto:

"The story is straightforward. We take it up at the time when Dr. Davidson abandoned his practice and professorship to give all his energies to research. That was 12 years ago. Davidson was convinced then that cancer was caused by changes within the body resulting from improper eating. 'Cancer is a nutritional deficiency disease,' he declared.

"This conclusion was derived from experiments on mice. Davidson found that the regular experimental forms of cancer could be produced easier in mice that had been raised on food lacking in vitamins. The opposite was also true. Mice fed special vitamin-rich diets were very resistant to cancer. Furthermore, after generations of mice were raised on vitamin-deficient diets, the offspring became more and more liable to cancer. In this Dr. Davidson believed that he had a clue to the puzzling fact that there are 'cancer susceptible' families, although the disease is definitely not hereditary.

"Linking the Davidson research with the virus theory, it could be said that the cancer virus, existing in bodies, passes over to the active, virulent form under certain definite chemical conditions brought about by prolonged lack of sufficient vitamins.

"Dr. Davidson was able to produce mice families susceptible to cancer. In five generations, by feeding with 'excess' vitamins and minerals, he bred from those susceptible mice a new generation quite free

[303]

CANCER: FACTS AND FALLACIES

from any abnormal tendency towards cancer. This type of evidence—the reversible demonstration—is among the most powerful that can be provided by experimental science.

"What are the vitamins used in the Davidson research? Mainly those associated with chicken embryos and with wheat germ. Why? Because the doctor's work convinced him that the disease of cancer is related in some way to normal cell multiplication that takes place so rapidly in developing embryos, such as that of the fertilized hen's egg. Here again there is nothing that is scientifically unsound.

"But it is from his clinical work that Dr. Davidson had collected most convincing evidence. He has stopped human cancer from spreading. He has completely cured some cases. A child suffering from lymphosarcoma and given only a few months to live was gradually restored to health without surgery or radium. After three years the affected glands were cured and normal.

"In this case the treatment consisted of special feeding. The Davidson diet is adjusted to individual patients, but in general includes large amounts of fresh vegetable juice (carrot and lettuce), raw vegetables (carrots, spinach, lettuce, peas, beans), wheat germ and rare beef. In addition, the patient gets massive doses of vitamins in the form of cod liver oil, wheat germ oil, and brewer's yeast. Finally there is a preparation made from chick embryos."

Dr. J. Ernest Ayre and Dr. W. A. G. Bould, of the Royal Victoria Hospital and McGill University, in

[304]

April, 1946, announced that they had discovered many cases of cancer that were due to vitamin deficiencies in the diet. Thye stated that there is "excellent circumstantial evidence to suggest that the nutritional deficiencies may have been a primary factor leading to the malignancy."

Dr. Arthur L. Wallace, a practicing physician for 45 years in Nashua, New Hampshire, appeared before the State Agricultural Advisory Board at Concord, New Hampshire on August 31, 1947, and said that, "if foodstuffs contained more nutrition, people would not be so susceptible to diseases such as cancer, heart ailments and other organic disorders. There appears to me to be too much seeking after disease-carrying germs these days, and then searching for wonder drugs to kill them off. It would be more beneficial if we corrected the nutritional deficiencies of the earth, and made people so healthy that they would not be susceptible to these same germs." He stated that "nutritional deficiency in the soil is the chief cause of increased diseases among people."

Sir Arbuthnot Lane, a famous English surgeon, has said: "Long surgical experience has proved to me conclusively that there is something radically and fundamentally wrong with the civilized mode of life, and I believe that unless the present dietetic and health customs of the white nations are recognized, social decay and race deterioration are inevitable."

I was amazed to read that the late Dr. Alexis Carrel in his classic "Man the Unknown" was aware of the dangers of using artificial fertilizers. In this book he

[305]

said: "Man is literally made from the dust of the earth. For this reason his physiological and mental activities are profoundly influenced by the geological constitution of the country where he lives, by the nature of the animals and plants on which he generally feeds. His structure and his functions depend also on the selections he makes of certain elements among the vegetal and animal foods at his disposal. The chiefs always had a diet quiet different from that of their slaves. Those who fought, commanded, and conquered used chiefly meats and fermented drinks, whereas the peaceful, the weak and the submissive were satisfied with milk, vegetables, fruits and cereals. Our aptitudes and our destiny come, in some measure, from the nature of the chemical substances that construct our tissues. It seems as though human beings, like animals, could be artificially given certain bodily and mental characteristics, if subjected from childhood to appropriate diets."

Carrel also remarks: "It (the organism) is also affected by the deficiencies of the essential physiological and mental functions. The staple foods may not contain the same nutritive substances as in former times. Mass production has modified the composition of wheat, eggs, milk, fruit, and butter, although these articles have retained their familiar appearance. Chemical fertilizers, by increasing the abundance of the crops without replacing all the exhausted elements of the soil, have indirectly contributed to change the nutritive value of cereal grains and of vegetables. Hens have been compelled by artificial diet and mode of

[306]

living, to enter the ranks of mass producers. Has not the quality of their eggs been modified? The same question may be asked about milk, because cows are now confined to the stable all year round, and are fed on manufactured provender. Hygienists have not paid sufficient attention to the genesis of diseases. Their studies of conditions of life and diet, and of their effects on the physiological and mental state of modern man, are superficial, incomplete, and of too short duration. . . ."

Dr. Carrel was also aware of the danger in placing too much confidence in the mortality statistics as a measure of our health. In this regard he said: "All diseases of bacterial origin have decreased in a striking manner. . . . But we still must die in a much larger proportion from degenerative diseases. In spite of the triumphs of medical science, the problem of disease is far from solved. Modern man is delicate; 1,100,000 persons have to attend the medical needs of 120,000,000 other persons. Every year, of this population in the United States, there are about 100,000,000 illnesses, serious or slight. In the hospitals, 700,000 beds are occupied every day of the year. . . . Medical care under all its forms, costs about $3,500,000,000 yearly. . . . The organism seems to have become more susceptible to degenerative diseases."

Now comes another physician of high standing, Dr. James Asa Shield, who at a convention of the Southern Medical Association on November 8, 1946, at Miami, Florida, attacked the use of chemical fertilizers in no uncertain terms. Let us quote from the Asso-

[307]

ciated Press dispatch which was sent across the wires of the country and which was printed in dozens of newspapers: "Dr. James Asa Shield, assistant professor of neuro-psychiatry of the Medical College of Virginia, said in an address before the Southern Medical Association convention here today that food produced from soil fertilized with chemicals has caused an increase of degenerative diseases throughout the United States.

"Shield charged that agriculture's attempt to correct soil exhaustion with chemicals has not been successful.

"The doctor must demand that the agriculturist produce a food that will meet the multiple cell needs for best growth, development and function," he said.

"Dr. Shield said one degenerative disease, multiple sclerosis, is virtually unknown in the Orient, where natural manures and plant refuse are used as fertilizers.

"He said the death rate from the disease in the United States is almost as high as the infantile paralysis death rate.

"Inorganic chemical fertilizers 'at times disturb the chemical balance of the soil and in turn affect the health of the animals that feed on the crops', the doctor reported.

"Despite deficiencies in vitamins, proteins and fats in the Chinese diet, they have no sclerosis of their nerves, their blood vessels, blockage of their veins or hypertension.

"He said several European countries that use chemical fertilizers have a high incidence of sclerosis and other degenerative diseases.

"The incomplete fertilization program carried on

[308]

in Europe and the United States is contributing largely to the inadequacy of the quality of the diet, with deficiency of minor minerals and unknown factors of this diet contributing to and being largely responsible for the presence of multiple sclerosis."

One of the greatest nutritionists of our time, Dr. E. V. McCollum of Johns Hopkins University, recently said, "When it comes to getting out of the soil and into the plant, elements which may be there already but which the plant cannot secure, the advocates of what is called the organic school of soil improvements have a good many persuasive arguments to present for their side of the case. Organic ferment may well stir up and release trace elements and other elements which commercial fertilizers alone can never provide." This quotation was given in a recent publication of *The Land* magazine.

The *American Journal of Digestive Diseases,* in its June, 1948 issue, referring to a book by N. Phillip Norman, M.D., and James Rorty, called *Tomorrow's Food,* said: "A careful study of the English authors who recommended natural compost for fertilizing purposes, particularly McCarrison and Howard, and of the experimental work of Maynard, Albrecht, Brody and others in this country, leaves one convinced of several facts. One fact is that until proper soil fertilization is practiced, we shall not be able to obtain from food (nor from artificial vitamins) the strongest known impetus to health. A second fact is that "where 'pedigreed' food products have been eaten under proper conditions of cooking, a most *amazing* degree of health

[309]

has been obtained both clinically and in experimental animals. It is not too much to say that such nutrition has been proved capable of *banishing disease of all kinds and of conferring a vigorous old age.* As Minot has recently indicated, the most important research today is nutritional research. Nobody knows the breadth, depth, or extent of the benefits in store for mankind as a result of the patient laborious efforts of our nutritional experts."

The *American Journal of Digestive Diseases* says further:

"Norman undoubtedly believes that 'proper' nutrition is capable of conferring upon an individual or a group, in due time, a superlative degree of fitness capable of relative immunity to infections and to the terrible degenerative changes so common now among older persons. . . . I think the best efforts of us all should be dedicated to what Norman has in mind. There are countless hurdles in the path. Vested interests will fold up only on public demand. Education alone can create a suitable public reaction. The *ideal of perfect nutrition* is the most dynamic concept before the profession today."

Dr. Norman was consulting nutritionist for the New York City Departments of Health and Hospitals.

I have to stop somewhere with these quotations from the thoughts of physicians. There are available dozens more. They show clearly that many physicians believe that there is some connection between the use of artificial fertilizers and the increasing incidence of cancer. Yet when one springs this concept upon a doctor who has not studied the subject he thinks you are crazy to think such a thing. Doctors must be made to think along the lines of good health coming from a soil rich in humus. They must set up experimental projects in which cancer cases in the early stages are fed on an exclusive diet of foods raised organically. In this respect I wish to state that the diets and foods given to patients in hospitals generally are atrocious—white breads, white sugars, canned foods.

There must arise special hospitals surrounded by their own farms which produce their own foods. In Canada there is one such hospital, an institution for the cure of mental cases. The medical superintendent of this hospital is Dr. F. H. E. Baugh, who enjoys a wide reputation as an authority on mental hygiene. Two farms totaling 400 acres are being conditioned by organic practices for the growing of the foods to be used in the Sanitarium. Dr. Baugh and his staff believe that organically grown foods rich in the essential vitamins and elements will greatly expedite the healing of sick minds. The building of the soil and the growing of the organic foods is under the supervision of J. D. Kennedy, bursar and secretary of the sanitarium, who is keenly interested in the relation between soil and health.

In the February, 1961, issue of the *American Journal of Proctology,* an extraordinary piece of research has been reported, which could revolutionize and simplify the whole concept of cancer. But before I comment on it, I should like to reproduce the entire article:

[311]

Anti-Malignancy Factors Apparently Present
in Organically-Grown Foods

By Donald D. Collins, M.D., F.I.A.P.

Hollywood, California

This clinical note is written with considerable hesitancy, and yet on five different occasions during the past 36 years of practice, I have seen a marvelous phenomenon occur.

Five patients have been observed with extensive malignancies, proven by biopsies, of either the gastrointestinal tract, or blood (leukemias), or sarcomas. Strangely, these five individuals all died many years later from diseases unrelated to these former malignant processes. It was shown in all five instances, following most thorough and painstaking autopsies, performed by highly competent pathologists, that no discernible pathologic evidence could be found then that such patients had ever previously had the various malignant diseases, proven by adequate biopsies to have been present in the past.

The only constant factor in the lives of these five persons was the fact that they all ate home raised, organically grown foods that were free from various chemical preservatives and insect repellent sprays. Unfortunately, here in Los Angeles we have learned to our dismay that smog apparently destroys these beneficial factor in organically grown foodstuffs. Possibly, such optimum foods possess unidentified antibiotic factors that are antagonistic to malignant growths in some humans. Some recent evidence attributes such beneficial actions to certain antibiotics studied so far.

This brief clinical note is written with the hope

[312]

CLINICAL CHART INVOLVING FIVE PATIENTS

Patient's Initials and Occupation	Sex, Age at Death, Race	Type of Malignancy and Grade	Metastases Present?	Age at Time of Diag. of Malig.	Location of Malig.	Was Surgery Performed?	Type of Operation Performed	Was Organically Grown Food Eaten? Pre-op.	Post op.
R. L. F. Painter	Male 84, White	Adeno Ca., iii.	Yes, in liver	52	Descend Colon	Yes	Partial Left—Colectomy Transverse to Sigmoid Colotomy.	No	Yes
S. R. S. Student, House-wife	Female 78, White	1. Osteogenic Saracoma, iii; 2. Adeno—Ca., ii.	1. ? 2. yes	1. $\frac{}{}$ 15, 2. $\frac{}{}$ 54	1. Rt. Femur, Mid.1/3; 2. Mid-rectum.	Yes	1. Amputation, Rt. Thigh Prox. 1/3 2. Comb. Abd.—Perineal Resection	1. No 2. No	1. No 2. Yes
J. R. McM. Butcher	Male 81, White	1. Adeno-Ca. kii 2. Lymph.—Ca, iii Leukemia 3. Adeno-Ca., iii.	1. Yes 2. Yes 3. Yes	1. 48 2. 50 3. 60	1. Stomach 2. Generalized 3. Recto-Sigmoid	1. Yes 2. Yes 3. Yes	1. 2/3 Gastric Resection, Ant. Polya. 2. Biopsy base L. Neck 3. Combin-Abd.—Perin. Resection	1. No 2. No 3. No	1. No 2. No 3. Yes
R. W. C. Janitor	Male 74, Negro	1. Hodgkins Disease	1. Yes 2. Yes	1. 27 2. 53	1. Gener-alized 2. Upper Rectum	1. Yes 2. Yes	1. Biopsy L. Axilla. 2. Comb. Abd.—Per-ineal Re-section	1. No 2. No	1. No 2. Yes
R. T. J. Accountant	Male 79, White	2. Adeno-Ca., iii.	Yes	59	Cecum	Yes	Rt. Hemi-Colectomy, Ileo-Trans-verse Colostomy	No	Yes

***Note:—These were all my own personal patients.

that it may prove of possible benefit to other colo-proctologists dealing with apparently hopeless malignant disease in their own patients. Surely, this recommended adjuvant therapy is innocuous and might prove life-prolonging or even arresting the further progress of malignant disease. This is certainly worth trying and remembering for possible future use.

This article appeared in February, 1961, and its contents should have been blared forth in the press. Yet not a word about it has been published in newspapers, magazines, or medical journals, other than where the original article was published. *Time* and *Newsweek,* which regularly comb medical journals for news on the medical front, failed to pick up this item. Perhaps this is due to the fact that orthodox medicine and the U. S. Government, as an official attitude, have characterized followers of the organic method as crackpots, cultists and food faddists.

The orthodox cancer-cure structure is such an elaborate setup with its billion dollar plant of hospitals, fancy treatment, x-ray machines, and other equipment, physicians, research men, technicians, etc., that it won't readily accept such a simple medicine—organically grown food—as a substitute. They will not stand by and see their impressive cancer edifice, with its millions of cancer fund income, collapse. They would lose face.

In the meantime, hundreds of thousands of people all over the world are dying and suffering from this dreadful disease, and no one bats an eyelash. In this

[314]

respect I must recall the amazing words of Dr. A. I. Lansing, the outgoing president of the Gerontological Society, who said on November 8, 1958, that finding a cure for cancer and heart disease would be a major financial disaster which would bankrupt the social security system and the big insurance companies. Is this why Dr. Collins' cancer cure results were not publicized?

We had a similar experience when there was published in November, 1949, the results of a feeding experiment with mice, sponsored by the Soil and Health Foundation of which I am president. The experiment was performed by Dr. Ehrenfried Pfeiffer at his Spring Valley, New York, laboratory. The results clearly showed that mice fed organically grown food suffered far less from cancer. Copies of the bulletin were sent to hundreds of medical journals and to the press, but none of them took any notice of it.

A doctor once said that cancer is Nature's revenge on man for living artificially. Eating organically grown food is living naturally. Eating chemically grown food full of chemical additives is living artificially and carries with it the possibility of getting cancer.

Anyone who has the smallest plot of soil should grow the vegetables for his family without using chemical fertilizers or poison sprays. Only composts and organic fertilizers and certain kinds of powdered rock should be used. It is not only insurance towards good health, but furnishes better-tasting food. And it is amazing how much food can be grown in a small plot. Besides, you will see creation before your very own eyes.

[315]

CHAPTER XXX

Which Path for Cancer Study?

Five years after a successful operation for breast cancer, a 35-year old mother of three remains a fugitive from society and reality: she will not let people see her, she blames the disease on herself, and she is besieged by feelings of anxiety, hostility, and depression. The surgical removal of her breast has cured her physically, but has it cured her mentally and emotionally?

An article by Professor Morton Bard in *Trans Action Magazine,* "The Price of Survival for Cancer Victims," (March-April, 1966, p. 10) points out that many cancer victims suffer from emotional anguish even after successful recovery. He cites cases of people who simply cannot adjust to the task of returning to a normal life with dignity and self-respect. The whole article raises the question of just how complete a cure surgery can ever be for cancer, since Professor Bard's research has found that successfully operated patients remain dreadfully sick in mind and in ability to live in society.

Certainly, research should be devoted to cures for existing cancers and to better methods of surgery. Yet, wouldn't it be much more rewarding to prevent cancer altogether, if that could be done? Some experiments by the Sloan-Kettering Institute for Cancer Research have shown that a healthy body can sometimes immunize itself against extracts from cancerous cells by producing antibodies to the foreign matter, and hence "rejecting" it. It would seem that the question for research is how to build and keep a body strong enough to resist disease. There is reason to believe that proper nutrition might play a vital role in preventing cancer.

Prevention Is Possible

Tests by Dr. Sugiura of The Sloan-Kettering Institute, have revealed that a diet supplemented with 15 per cent brewer's yeast and 10 per cent desiccated liver prevented liver cancer in rats fed a cancer-producing food additive—butter yellow. In addition, a report presented by Dr. George S. Sharp to the James Ewing Society (April 2, 1959) indicated that patients with precancerous lesions of the oral mucous membranes improved greatly with supplements of desiccated liver, vitamin B_{12}, riboflavin (B_2), folic acid (a B complex vitamin found in raw vegetables), plus a diet designed not to aggravate any further soreness of the mouth. Thirty out of 34 patients improved so much that they could wear dentures comfortably for 24 hours, whereas before nutritional care, they had low tolerance for

[317]

CANCER: FACTS AND FALLACIES

dentures. We might heed a statement from Dr. Sharp himself: "In cancer control, prophylaxis has been one of the least investigated among the various therapeutic measures tried. However, in oral cancer, definite studies are showing that precancerous conditions can be returned to normal."

Encouraging as these results are, far more research is needed to learn just what is responsible for immunizing the entire body, not only localized organs, against disease and how this immunity can be encouraged and increased. One group of people, the Hunzas of India, appear totally resistant to many diseases, including cancer. Because they are economically poor and isolated, they have no access to sugar and grain refineries, tin cans, and the food processes American companies perform—flavoring, coloring, denaturing, and preserving. The Hunzas eat their fruits and vegetables raw, with skins. Because of a food scarcity, they do not have much of a chance to become overweight. They live in fresh air and sunlight, and do not use chemical fertilizers in their soil.

Refined Food Clue

What do these habits tell us about a healthy people and about ourselves? In a book by T. L. Cleave, a surgeon captain in Britain, entitled *Diabetes, Coronary Thrombosis, and the Saccharine Disease,* an interesting theory blames refined carbohydrates, such as white flour and white or brown sugar, for the many ailments encountered by Western civilization. The author states, "Refining by machinery is so recent a practice that we are not adapted to it at all. . . ." He also suggests that ". . . of all the foods that exhibit an alteration from the natural state, the refined carbohydrates . . . exhibit the greatest." Studying these facts, might we not consider environmental conditions (including nutrition) as affecting resistance? In the United States, most of us eat refined pastries and candies, breathe in polluted air, drink impure water, weigh a little too much, overcook our food, and get sick at least a few times in our lives.

From this brief comparison of primitive and "civilized" living, we cannot conclusively state that simple eating definitely prevents cancer. Yet, there is the fact of what we do to our foods before we eat them. In most cases, we do not receive the full value from nutrients that we should. We have come away from "nature's way" to "man's way" through canning, coloring, etc.

One more instance of our habit of altering food is the process of smoking meats. In Iceland and in Baltic areas, Dr. Kraybill of the National Cancer Institute received a report that fishermen who ate smoked fish had a three times higher incidence of cancer than those who lived inland. These fishermen eating smoked fish had a rate of gastrointestinal cancer four times that of populations not eating smoked fish. Stomach cancer in these countries accounted for 35 per cent to 45 per cent of all malignant tumors.

So far, then, it seems that we are digging our own graves by the way we eat. Yet, current research is not conclusive enough to tell us exactly what foods to improve, avoid, or add. There are many hints, but not enough specific answers. Nutrition is the one area that affects all of us because we all must eat. If cancer-immunizing procedures are to be effective, our bodies must first be strong. The search for cancer cures is full of good intentions, but disease is a case of good health turned poor.

Since "we are what we eat," it seems only reasonable that investigation should follow up the exact effects of all foods on cells. For instance, it might be wise to study the influences of calcium and magnesium, since some theories suggest that cancer spreads because of deficiencies of these elements in the cell. Oxygen might also be another factor in preventing abnormal cell formations. Very hot beverages might be responsible for irritating the esophagus. *World Health Magazine* has found a link between obese people and gall bladder cancer. All of these areas demand intensive investigation if we are to be rid of this dread disease for ever. Is such a dream possible? The signs say yes, but first we need more proofs; only then can a system of prevention take place.

The final answer to a cure for cancer lies in its prevention. Let us hope that funds allocated by the Public Health Service will be channelled toward promoting immunity and resistance, rather than "cures" which heal the body but leave the soul sick.

[320]

Index

[321]

Date Due